INTERMITTENT FASTING 16/8

DIET COOKBOOK

This Diet Recipe Cookbook Belongs To:

_____

TABLE OF CONTENTS

1. **INTRODUCTION**
2. **30 DELICIOUS AND HEALTHY COOKBOOK RECIPES**
3. **CONCLUSION**

INTRODUCTION

Intermittent Fasting refers to dietary eating patterns that involve not eating or severely restricting calories for a prolonged period of time. There are many different subgroups of intermittent fasting each with individual variation in the duration of the fast; some for hours, others for the day(s). This has become an extremely popular topic in the science community due to all of the potential benefits on fitness and health that are being discovered.

Types Of Intermittent Fasting:

Intermittent fasting comes in various forms and each may have a specific set of unique benefits. Each form of intermittent fasting has variations in the fasting-to-eating ratio. The benefits and effectiveness of these different protocols may differ on an individual basis and it is important to determine which one is best for you. Factors that may influence which one to choose include health goals, daily schedule/routine, and current health status. The most common types of Intermittent Fasting are alternate day fasting, time-restricted feeding, and modified fasting.

1. Alternate Day Fasting:

This approach involves alternating days of absolutely no calories (from food or beverage) with days of free feeding and eating whatever you want.

This plan has been shown to help with weight loss, improve blood cholesterol and triglyceride (fat) levels, and improve markers for inflammation in the blood.

The main downfall with this form of intermittent fasting is that it is the most difficult to stick with because of the reported hunger during fasting days.

2. Modified Fasting - 5:2 Diet

Modified fasting is a protocol with programmed fasting days, but the fasting days do allow for some food intake. Generally, 20-25% of normal calories are allowed to be consumed on fasting days; so if you normally consume 2000 calories on regular eating days, you would be allowed 400-500 calories on fasting days. The 5:2 part of this diet refers to the ratio of non-fasting to fasting days. So on this regimen, you would eat normally for 5 consecutive days, then fast or restrict calories to 20-25% for 2 consecutive days.

This protocol is great for weight loss, body composition, and may also benefit the regulation of blood sugar, lipids, and inflammation. Studies have shown the 5:2 protocol to be effective for weight loss, improve/lower inflammation markers in the blood (3), and show signs trending improvements in insulin resistance. In animal studies, this modified fasting 5:2 diet resulted in decreased fat, decreased hunger hormones (leptin), and increased levels of a protein responsible for improvements in fat burning and blood sugar regulation (adiponectin).

The modified 5:2 fasting protocol is easy to follow and has a small number of negative side effects which included hunger, low energy, and some irritability when beginning the program. Contrary to this, however, studies have also noted improvements such as reduced tension, less anger, less fatigue, improvements in self-confidence, and a more positive mood.

3. Time-Restricted Feeding:

If you know anyone that has said they are doing intermittent fasting, odds are it is in the form of time-restricted feeding. This is a type of intermittent fasting that is used daily and it involves only consuming calories during a small portion of the day and fasting for the remainder. Daily fasting intervals in time-restricted feeding may range from 12-20 hours, with the most common method being 16/8 (fasting for 16 hours, consuming calories for 8). For this protocol, the time of day is not important as long as you are fasting for a consecutive period of time and only eating in your allowed time period. For example, on a 16/8 time-restricted feeding program one person may eat their first meal at 7 AM and last meal at 3 PM (fast from 3PM-7AM), while another person may eat their first meal at 1 PM and last meal at 9 PM (fast from 9PM-1PM). This protocol is meant to be performed every day over long periods of time and is very flexible as long as you are staying within the fasting/eating window(s).

Time-Restricted feeding is one of the easiest to follow methods of intermittent fasting. Using this along with your daily work and sleep schedule may help achieve optimal metabolic function. Time-restricted feeding is a great program to follow for weight loss and body composition improvements as well as some other overall health benefits. The few human trials that were conducted noted significant reductions in weight, reductions in fasting blood glucose, and improvements in cholesterol with no changes in perceived tension, depression, anger, fatigue, or confusion. Some other preliminary results from animal studies showed time-restricted feeding to protect against obesity, high insulin levels, fatty liver disease, and inflammation.

The easy application and promising results of time-restricted feeding could possibly make it an excellent option for weight loss and chronic disease prevention/management. When implementing this protocol it may be good, to begin with, a lower fasting-to-eating ratio like 12/12 hours and eventually work your way up to 16/8 hours.

Many fitness clinics and nutritionists advocate this method to achieve a healthy lifestyle. Fasting for 2 days (not consecutive) and then eating whatever you like for the other 5 days of the week is a very interesting diet plan for everyone wishing to lose weight and/or have a healthy life.

There Are Many Benefits To This Plan.

- The main advantage gained for weight loss by this type of fasting is longer life expectancy by a change of diets. By having a diet plan everyone worldwide can benefit from intermittent fasting and lose weight

- A recent case study showed that people who fast recurrently live about 40% longer than the average life span of people in the same country; although this is very difficult to believe.
- Intermittent fasting reduces the risk of diabetes, cancer, and hypertension.
- Diabetes, cancer, and hypertension are among the most life-threatening diseases all over the world causing thousands of deaths each year.
- Moderated fasting will assist in protecting you from these chronic diseases.
- Fasting also is a great detoxifier of your body tissues.
- It is imperative that a diet plan is strictly adhered to so that your system gets sufficient rest and all harmful particles of the body are removed.
- This process is known as a natural cleansing and will restore the natural balance in all major systems of the body.
- Improved fitness and weight loss are the two biggest attractions for intermittent fasting.
- By going on a course of such dieting will go a long way to arriving at your desired body weight.
- This fasting method is widely used and is a safe and proven method of weight loss. If, however, you are pregnant it should not be used.
- You will burn off all excessive pounds of fat making you physically fitter.
- Healthy young adults will normally gain most from it.
- It is important that if you believe you have a major health problem you should see a doctor first to ensure that it is safe to go on such a fasting course.
- Always allow your body to absorb the changes over several steps.
- This will ensure you will keep fit and healthy and safe from any unwanted effects.

In this eBook, you will find quick and easy, Delicious and Healthy Cookbook Recipes, With Easy to Follow Instructions for Intermittent fasting.

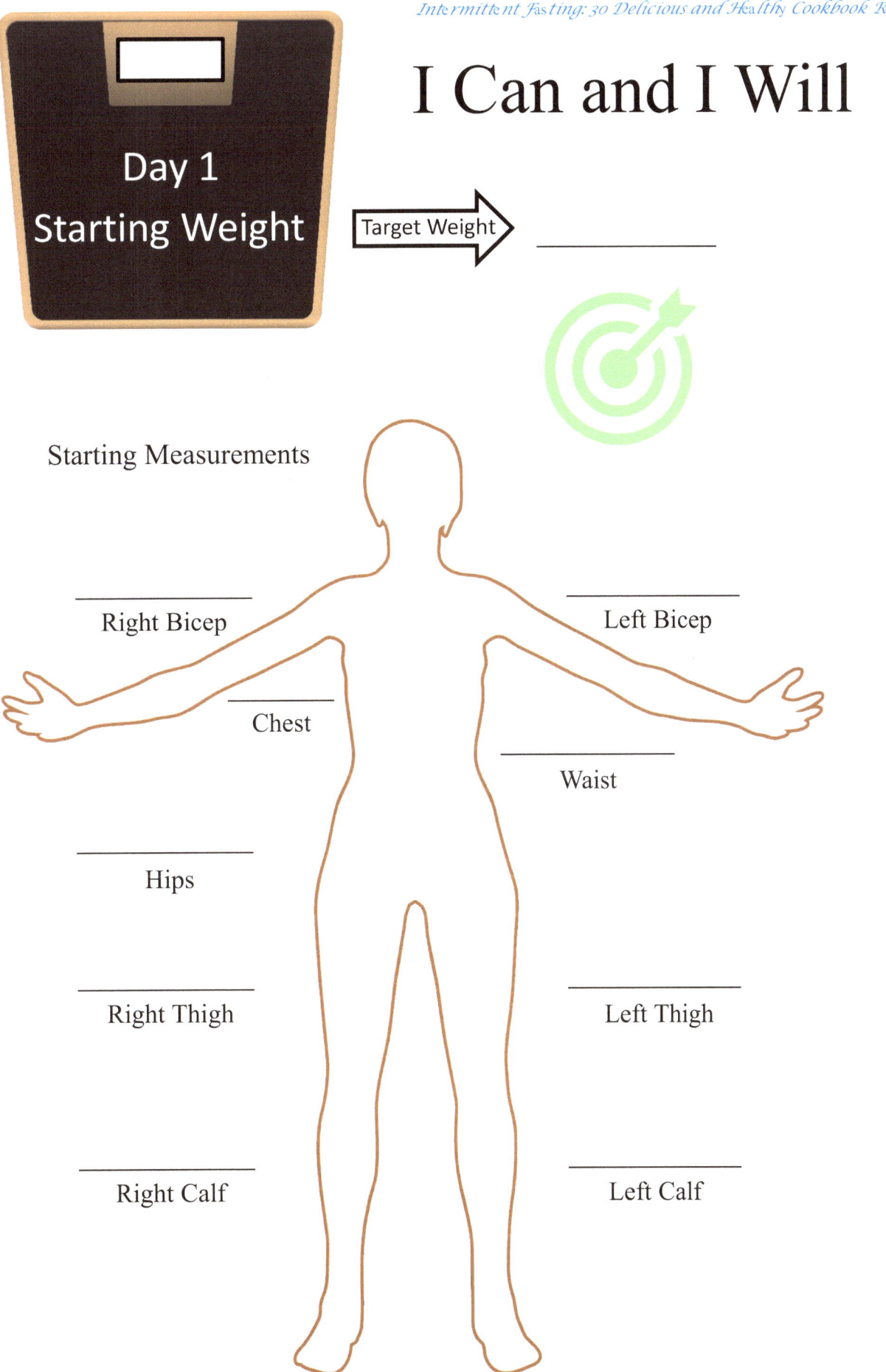

Intermittent Fasting: 30 Delicious and Healthy Cookbook Recipes

INTERMITTENT FASTING RECIPES

1. AVOCADO EGG SALAD

Prep Time: 15 mins Total Time: 15 mins

Servings: 4

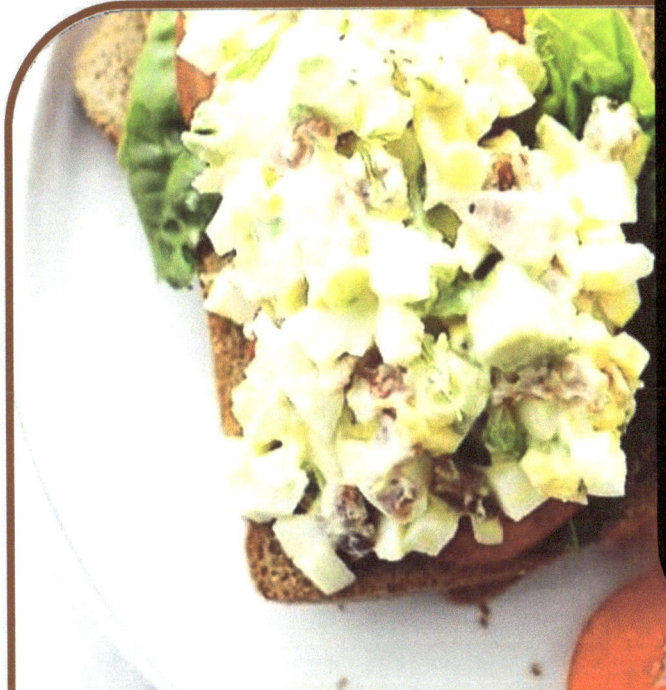

Ingredients
- 4 large hard-boiled eggs, diced
- 1 avocado, diced
- 2 green onions, sliced into thin rounds
- 4 slices of low-sodium bacon, cooked to the desired crisp and crumbled
- 1/4- cup nonfat plain yogurt
- 1 tablespoon low-fat sour cream
- 1 whole lime, juiced
- 1 tablespoon snipped fresh dill
- 1/4 teaspoon salt
- 1/8 teaspoon fresh ground pepper
- dill and crumbled bacon, for garnish (optional)

Directions:

1. To "boil" eggs, place each egg in the cavity of a muffin tin and hard "boil" in the oven for 30 minutes at 325F.
2. Remove from oven and transfer eggs to ice water; peel and dice.
3. In a salad bowl, combine diced eggs, avocado, green onions, and bacon; set aside.
4. In a mixing bowl, whisk together yogurt, sour cream, lime juice, dill, salt, and pepper; whisk until well combined.
5. Add yogurt mixture to the egg salad; stir until combined.
6. Garnish with dill and crumbled bacon.
7. Serve.
8. You can also spread the salad on 4 slices of bread; add tomatoes and lettuce to make a delicious egg salad sandwich.
9. Keep refrigerated.

2. SMOKEY GREEN BEAN TURKEY SKILLET

Prep Time: 5 minutes Cook Time: 15 minutes
Total Time: 20 minutes

Servings: 4

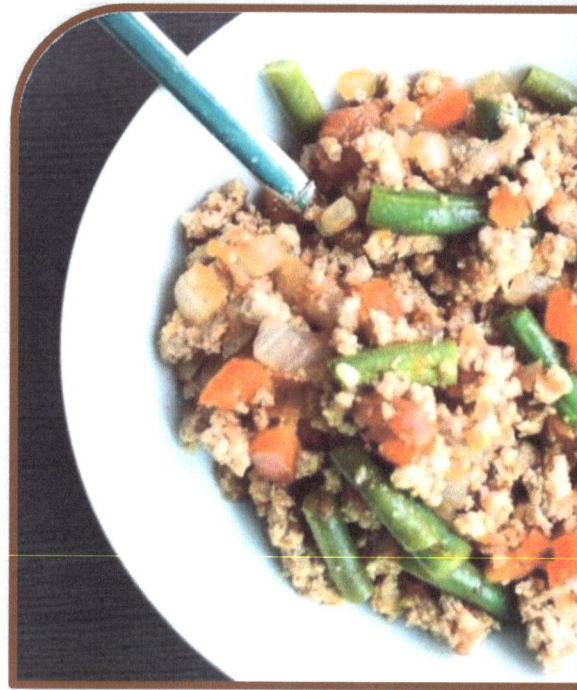

Ingredients

- 1 tablespoon olive oil (or avo oil)
- 1pound lean ground turkey
- 1/2 teaspoon garlic, minced
- 1 red bell pepper, diced
- 1/2 yellow onion, diced
- 2cups fresh green beans, ends removed, cut into 1 or 2-inch lengths (about 8 oz)
- 2 teaspoons smoke seasoning blend (see note for alternatives)
- 3/4 cup chipotle salsa (any salsa will work)
- pinch of salt
- Optional: serve with rice, quinoa, pasta, greens

Directions:

1. Heat olive oil in a large skillet over medium-high heat. Add ground turkey and break apart with a spatula. Add a pinch of salt. Cook until meat is nearly cooked through, about 4-5 minutes. Remove excess liquid from pan.
2. Push turkey meat to one side of the skillet. Add red pepper, onion, green beans, and garlic. Mix meat and vegetables together and sauté for 3-4 more minutes, stirring occasionally.
3. Add seasoning and salsa. Mix ingredients in the skillet until evenly distributed. Reduce heat to low, and simmer for 6-7 minutes or until green beans are tender, stirring occasionally.
4. Serve over rice, quinoa, or pasta! Store in an airtight container in the refrigerator for up to 4 days.

3. CHICKEN AND BROCCOLI STIR FRY

Prep Time 10 minutes Cook Time 20 minutes
Total Time 30 minutes

Servings: 4

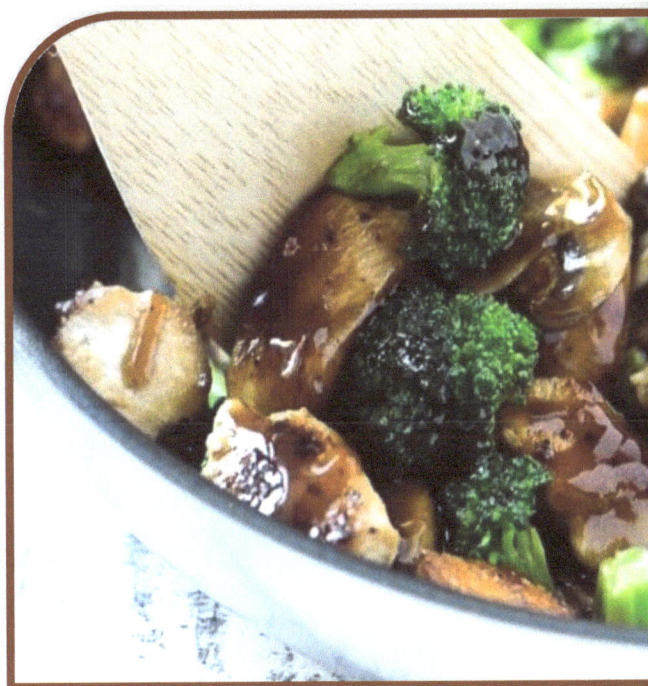

Ingredients

- 1 pound boneless skinless chicken breast cut into 1 inch pieces
- 1 tablespoon + 1 teaspoon vegetable oil
- 2 cups small broccoli florets
- 3 cup sliced mushrooms if you don't like mushrooms you can add more broccoli instead
- 4 teaspoons minced fresh ginger
- 1 teaspoon minced garlic
- 1/4 cup oyster sauce
- 1/4 cup low sodium chicken broth or water
- 1 teaspoon sugar
- 2 teaspoons toasted sesame oil
- 1 teaspoon soy sauce
- 1 teaspoon cornstarch
- salt and pepper to taste

Directions:

1. Heat 1 teaspoon of oil in a large frying pan over medium heat.
2. Add the broccoli and mushrooms and cook for approximately 4 minutes or until vegetables are tender.
3. Add the ginger and garlic to the pan and cook for 30 seconds more.
4. Remove the vegetables from the pan; place them on a plate and cover.
5. Wipe the pan clean with a paper towel and turn the heat to high. Add the remaining tablespoon of oil.
6. Season the chicken pieces with salt and pepper and add them to the pan in a single layer - you may need to do this step in batches. Cook for 3-4 minutes on each side until golden brown and cooked through.
7. Add the vegetables back to the pan and cook for 2 more minutes or until the vegetables are warmed through.
8. In a bowl whisk together the oyster sauce, chicken broth, sugar, sesame oil, and soy sauce. In a small bowl mix the cornstarch with a tablespoon of cold water.
9. Pour the oyster sauce mixture over the chicken and vegetables; cook for 30 seconds. Add the cornstarch and bring to a boil; cook for 1 more minute or until the sauce has just started to thicken.
10. Serve immediately, with rice if desired.

4. QUICK AND EASY PALEO EGG MUFFINS RECIPE

Prep Time: 20 minutes Cook Time: 20 minutes

Total Time: 40 minutes

Servings: 12

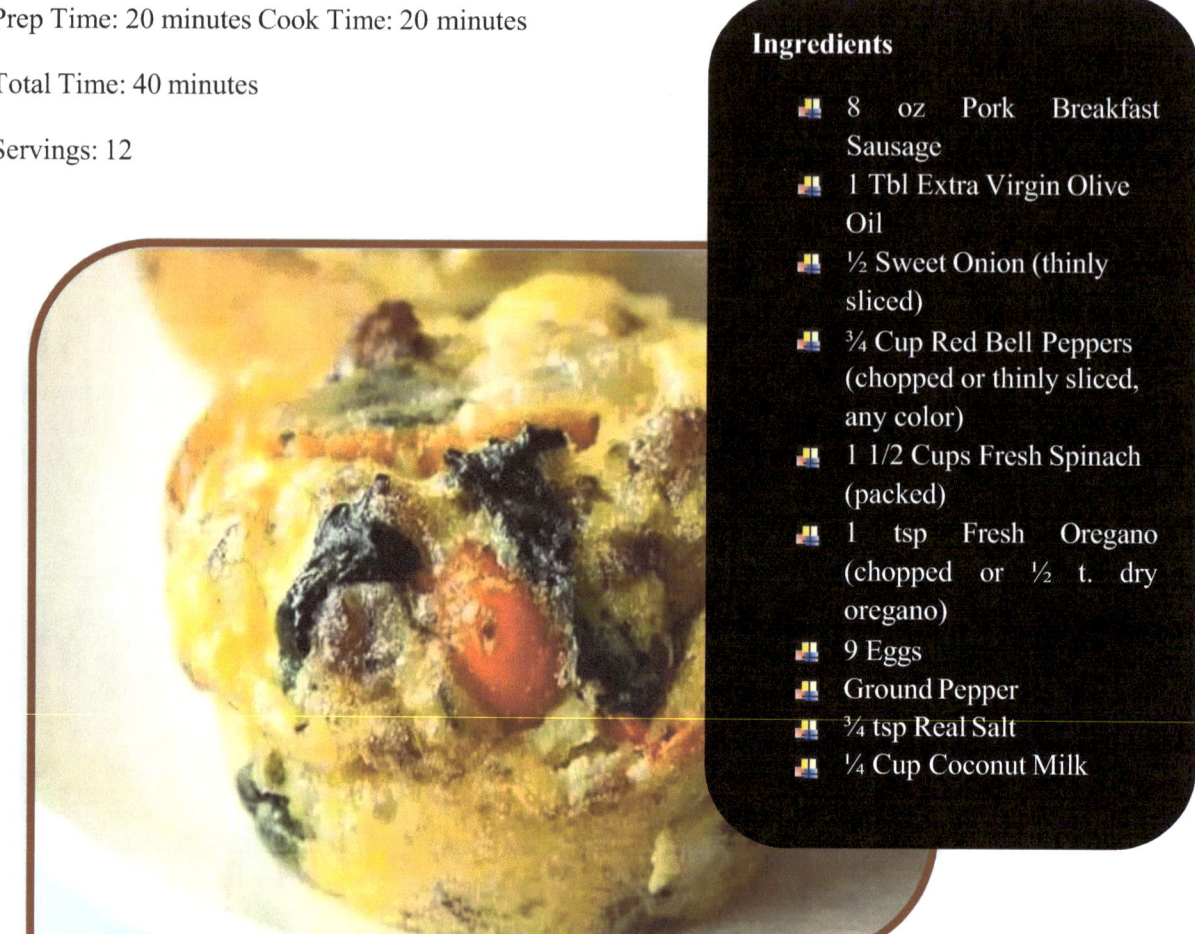

Ingredients
- 8 oz Pork Breakfast Sausage
- 1 Tbl Extra Virgin Olive Oil
- ½ Sweet Onion (thinly sliced)
- ¾ Cup Red Bell Peppers (chopped or thinly sliced, any color)
- 1 1/2 Cups Fresh Spinach (packed)
- 1 tsp Fresh Oregano (chopped or ½ t. dry oregano)
- 9 Eggs
- Ground Pepper
- ¼ tsp Real Salt
- ¼ Cup Coconut Milk

Directions:

1. Preheat oven to 350 degrees. Grease a muffin tin.
2. Place the ground sausage in a sauté pan and heat on medium high. Break up the pork into crumbles with a spatula as it cooks.
3. When the pork is halfway cooked, add 1 T. of olive oil, onions, peppers, and oregano to the pan. Sauté until the onion is translucent. Add the spinach to the pan and cover with a lid. Cook for 30 seconds, remove the lid and toss the ingredients. Spinach should be wilted but still bright green. Remove from heat.
4. Place the eggs in a large mixing bowl along with the pepper, salt, and milk. Whisk together until eggs are well beaten.
5. Add the sausage and vegetables to the egg mixture and mix in until well distributed.
6. Divide the mixture between the greased muffin tins(12 total), making sure that each tin has a somewhat equal ratio of eggs/fillings.
7. Bake in preheated oven for 18-20 minutes. Cool for a few minutes and remove from tins, loosening the edges first with a knife.

5. PORK EGG ROLL IN A BOWL

Prep Time: 5 minutes Cook Time: 25 minutes

Total Time: 30 minutes

Servings: 4

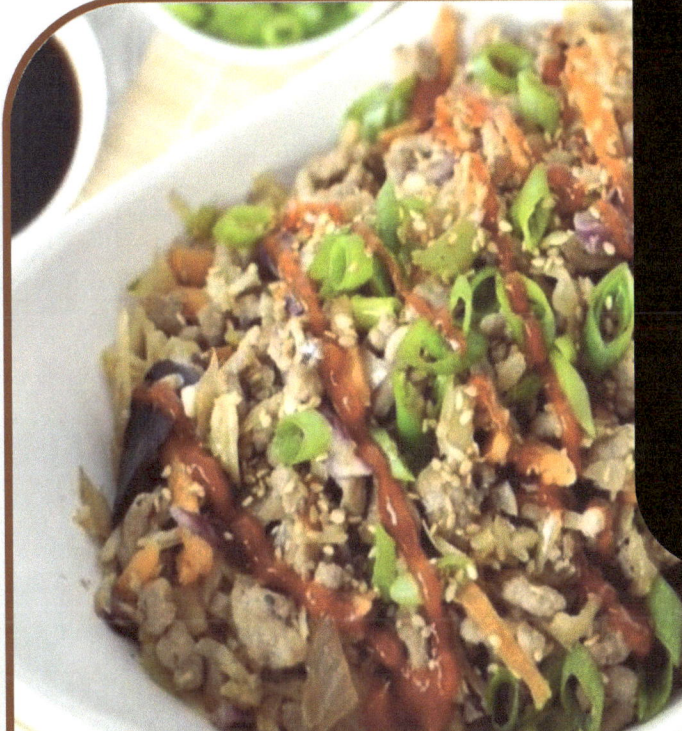

Ingredients

- 2 tablespoons sesame oil
- 3 cloves garlic, minced
- 1/2 cup onion, diced
- 5 green onions, sliced on a bias (white and green parts)
- 1 pound ground pork
- 1/2 teaspoon ground ginger
- sea salt and black pepper, to taste
- 1 tablespoon Sriracha or garlic chili sauce, more to taste
- 14-ounce bag coleslaw mix
- 3 tablespoons Coconut Aminos or gluten-free soy sauce
- 1 tablespoon rice vinegar
- 2 tablespoons toasted sesame seeds

Directions:

1. Heat sesame oil in a large skillet over medium-high heat.
2. Add the garlic, onion, and white portion of the green onions.
3. Sauté until the onions are translucent and the garlic is fragrant.
4. Add the ground pork, ground ginger, sea salt, black pepper, and Sriracha. Sauté until the pork is cooked through.
5. Add the coleslaw mix, coconut aminos, and rice wine vinegar.
6. Sauté until the coleslaw is tender.
7. Top with green onions and sesame seeds before serving.

6. GLUTEN FREE, LOW CARB & KETO FISH TACOS

Prep Time: 20 minutes Cook Time: 15 minutes
Marinating Time: 2 hours
Servings: 4

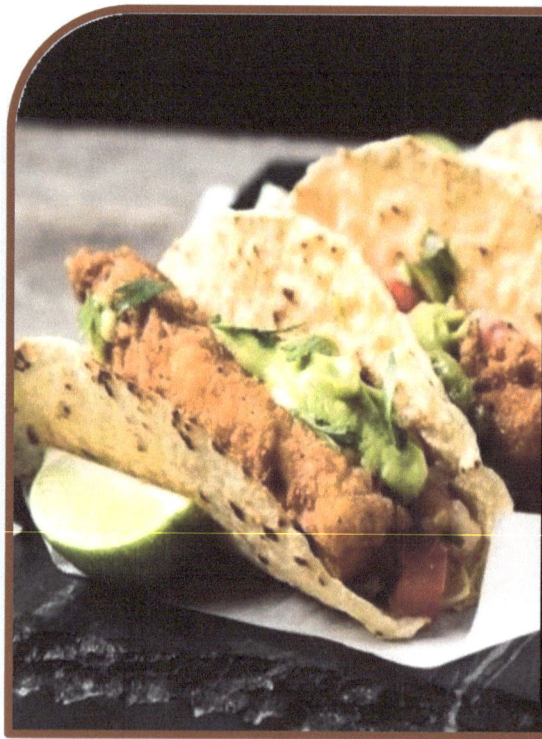

Ingredients

For the gluten free & Keto fish tacos
- 250 g firm white-flesh fish such as flounder or cod
- 1/3 cup sour cream or coconut cream + 2 tsp apple cider vinegar
- 2 teaspoons apple cider vinegar
- 4 cloves garlic ran through a press
- kosher salt to taste
- 1/2 cup whey protein isolate
- 1 teaspoon baking powder
- 1 1/2 teaspoon chili powder
- 1/4-1/2 teaspoon kosher salt to taste
- 1 egg
- 1 tablespoon sour cream or coconut cream
- 2 teaspoons apple cider vinegar
- coconut oil or cooking oil of choice

Serving suggestions
- 1 batch 15-minute Keto & grain free tortillas 8 tortillas
- 1 batch pico de gallo salsa
- guacamole

Directions:
1. Mix sour (or coconut) cream, vinegar, garlic and season to taste with salt. Cut the fish across the grain of the flesh into strips roughly 1/2 inch wide, and add it to the cream marinade. Cover and refrigerate for two hours, preferably overnight.
2. Make a batch of our grain free Keto tortillas. You can have them shaped and ready to go for cooking them simultaneously to the fish.
3. Prepare your frying station by adding enough oil to a skillet or pan to make it about 1/2-inch deep. You can save a lot of oil by using a narrower pan and frying in batches. Heat up oil over medium/low heat while you coat the fish.
4. Mix the whey protein, baking powder, chili powder and salt in a shallow plate or dish. In a second plate or dish, whisk the egg with cream and vinegar.
5. Coat the fish by lightly removing excess marinade, dipping in the egg mix, followed by the whey protein mix, immediately placing in the hot oil and basting the top right away. You want to fry the fish right after coating for best crispness. Fry on both sides until deep golden and transfer to a paper-lined plate for a couple of minutes.
6. Serve right away with the freshly-made tortillas, plenty of limes and your salsa of choice.

7. CUMIN SPICED BEEF WRAPS

Prep Time: 15 mins Cook Time: 10 mins Total Time: 25 mins

Servings: 2

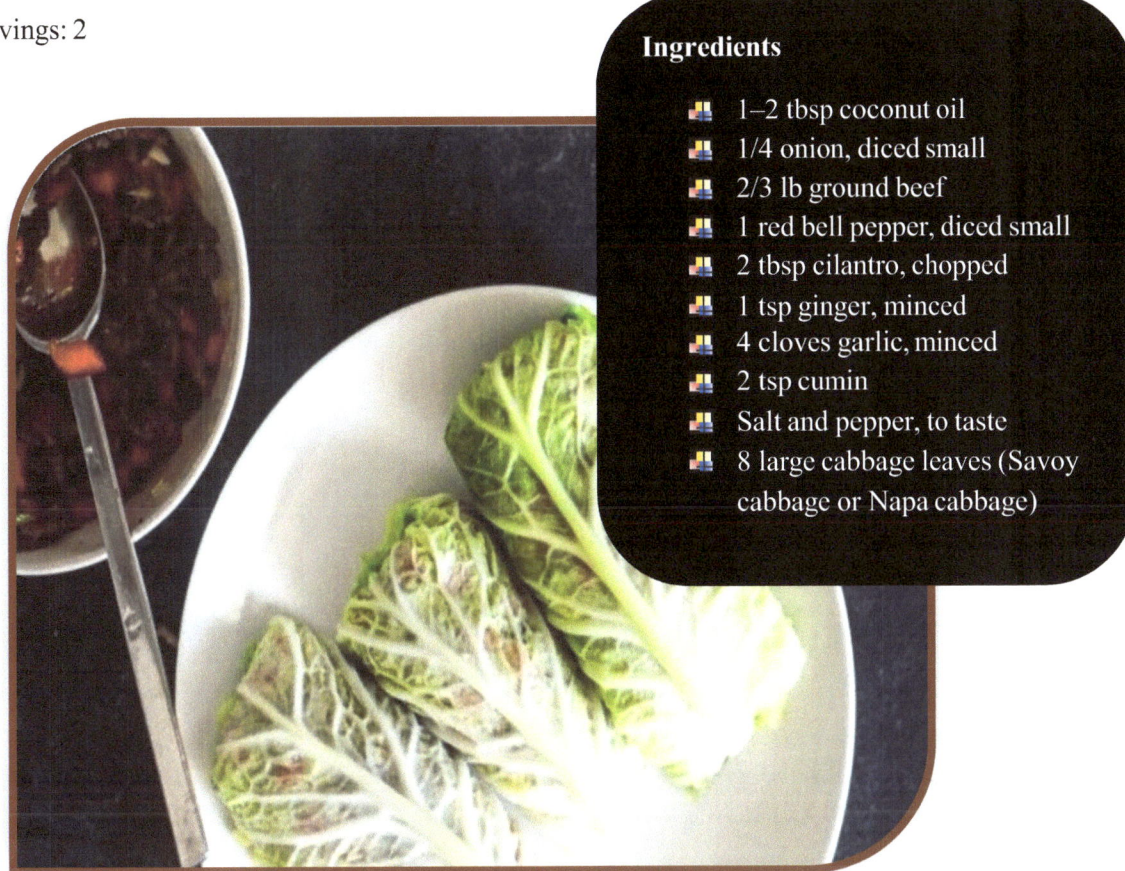

Ingredients

- 1–2 tbsp coconut oil
- 1/4 onion, diced small
- 2/3 lb ground beef
- 1 red bell pepper, diced small
- 2 tbsp cilantro, chopped
- 1 tsp ginger, minced
- 4 cloves garlic, minced
- 2 tsp cumin
- Salt and pepper, to taste
- 8 large cabbage leaves (Savoy cabbage or Napa cabbage)

Directions:

1. Place 1-2 tbsp of coconut oil into a frying pan and sauté the onions, ground beef, and peppers on medium heat.
2. When the ground beef is cooked, add in the cilantro, ginger, garlic, cumin, salt, and pepper to taste.
3. Fill a large pot 3/4 full with water and bring to a boil.
4. Using tongs, blanch each cabbage leaf in the boiling water (put each leaf into the boiling water for 20 seconds). Then plunge each leaf into some cold water before draining and placing onto a plate.
5. Spoon the beef mixture onto each lettuce leaf and fold into a roll.

8. HEALTHY FLUFFY LOW CARB PANCAKES

Prep Time: 10 mins Cook Time: 5 mins Total Time: 15 mins

Servings: 2

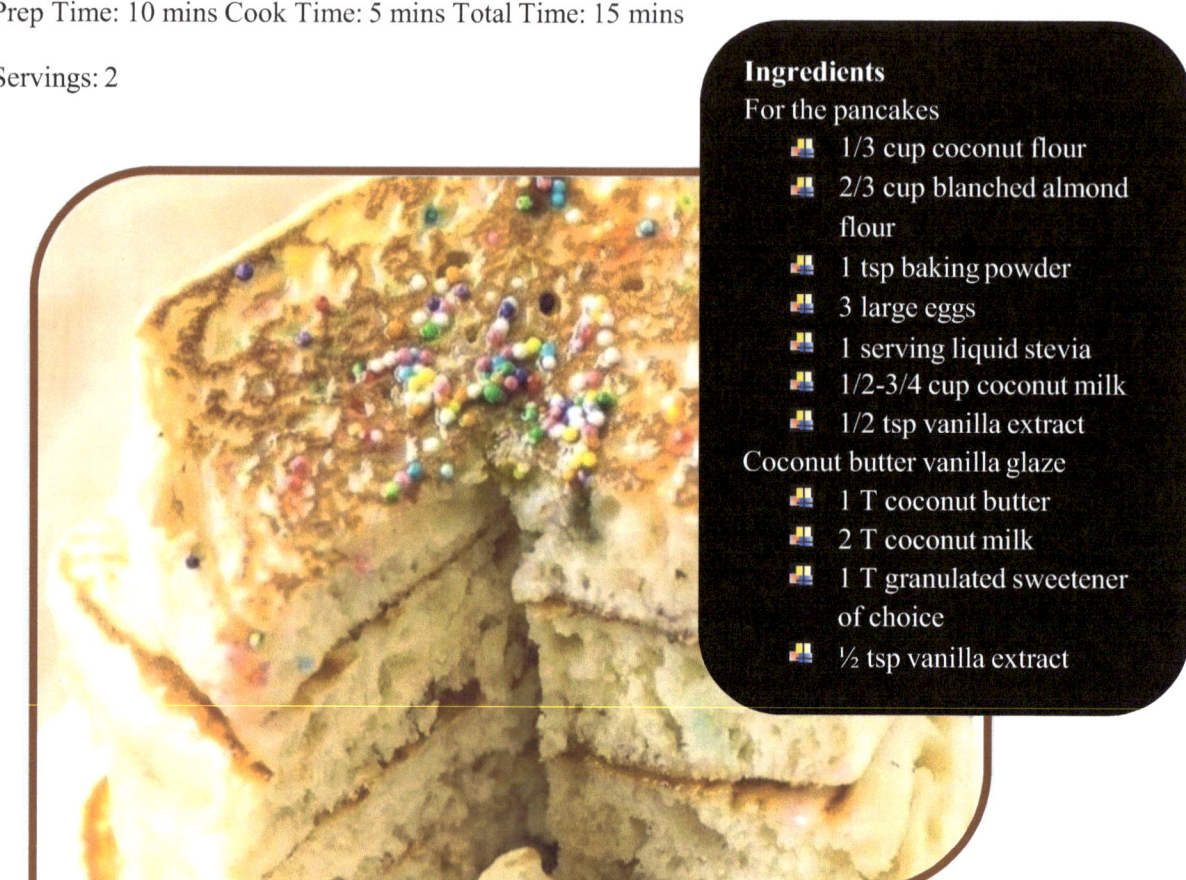

Ingredients
For the pancakes
- 1/3 cup coconut flour
- 2/3 cup blanched almond flour
- 1 tsp baking powder
- 3 large eggs
- 1 serving liquid stevia
- 1/2-3/4 cup coconut milk
- 1/2 tsp vanilla extract

Coconut butter vanilla glaze
- 1 T coconut butter
- 2 T coconut milk
- 1 T granulated sweetener of choice
- ½ tsp vanilla extract

Directions:

1. In a large mixing bowl, add your dry ingredients and set aside.
2. In two small bowls, separate the egg yolks from the whites.
3. Add the egg yolks, coconut milk, and liquid stevia to the dry ingredients and mix very well. If the batter is too thin, add the extra almond flour. If the batter is too thick, thin it out with a little extra coconut milk.
4. Whisk the egg whites well, until slight peaks start to form.
5. Slowly fold into the pancake batter and allow to sit to thicken approximately 5 minutes.
6. Grease a non-stick pan on medium heat. When hot, pour small 1/4 cup portions of the batter and if possible, place a lid on top.
7. When bubbles start to form on the edges, flip and continue cooking until slightly golden. Repeat until all the pancake batter is used up.
8. Prepare your optional glaze by combining all your ingredients and drizzling over the cooked pancakes.

9. LOW CARB CHICKEN ZUCCHINI ENCHILADA BAKE

Prep time: 15 mins Cook time: 30 mins
Total time: 45 mins
Servings: 6

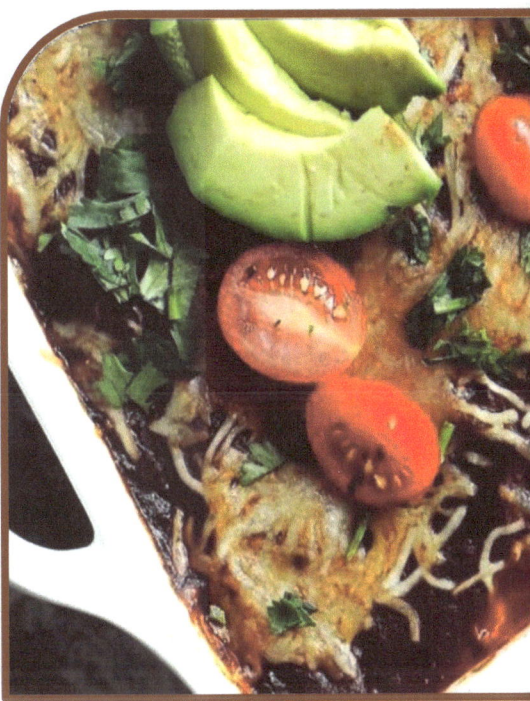

Ingredients

Homemade Enchilada Sauce:
- 2 teaspoons olive oil
- 1 small white onion, finely diced
- 3 cloves garlic, minced
- 2 1/2 tablespoons chili powder
- 1 teaspoon cumin
- 1 teaspoon dried oregano
- 1/4 teaspoon salt
- 1- 15 oz can tomato sauce
- 2 tablespoons tomato paste
- 1/2 cup water (or broth of choice)
- 1/2 teaspoon apple cider vinegar
- Salt and pepper, to taste

For the casserole:
- 2 large zucchini, cut lengthwise into 1/8" thick slices
- 1 cup refried beans
- 2 cups shredded, cooked chicken breast
- 1 small white onion, diced
- 1 medium red bell pepper, chopped
- 1 cup fresh or frozen sweet corn
- 1 1/2 cups Go Veggie Cheddar Shreds or regular shredded

Directions:

1. Make enchilada sauce: Heat oil in a medium pot over medium-high heat. Add in onions and garlic and sauté for 5 minutes or until onions become translucent. Add in chili powder, cumin, oregano, salt and stir for 30 seconds to allow the spices to cook a bit. Stir in tomato sauce, tomato paste, water, and apple cider vinegar then bring to a boil. Reduce heat to low and simmer for about 5-10 minutes. Season with additional salt and pepper to taste, if necessary. Makes about 2 cups of enchilada sauce
2. Preheat oven to 350 degrees F.
3. Add 1/2 cup enchilada sauce to the bottom of a 9x9 inch pan coated with nonstick cooking spray. Place zucchini slices evenly over sauce to cover and create a single layer. Next spread half of the refried beans (you may need to warm them to help spread), half of the shredded chicken, half of the corn, half the onion, and half the pepper, and 1/2 cup cheese. Repeat layers again, starting with remaining enchilada sauce, zucchini slices, refried beans, chicken, corn, onion, red pepper, and 1/2 cup cheese. Top with any remaining enchilada sauce, then finishing with 1/2 cup cheese.
4. Bake for 30 minutes covered with foil, then remove the cover and bake another 10-15 minutes. Top with jalapenos, cilantro, greek yogurt, and hot sauce, if desired!

10. RED MULLET WITH BAKED TOMATOES

Prep Time: less than 30 mins Cooking Time: 10-30 mins

Servings: 4

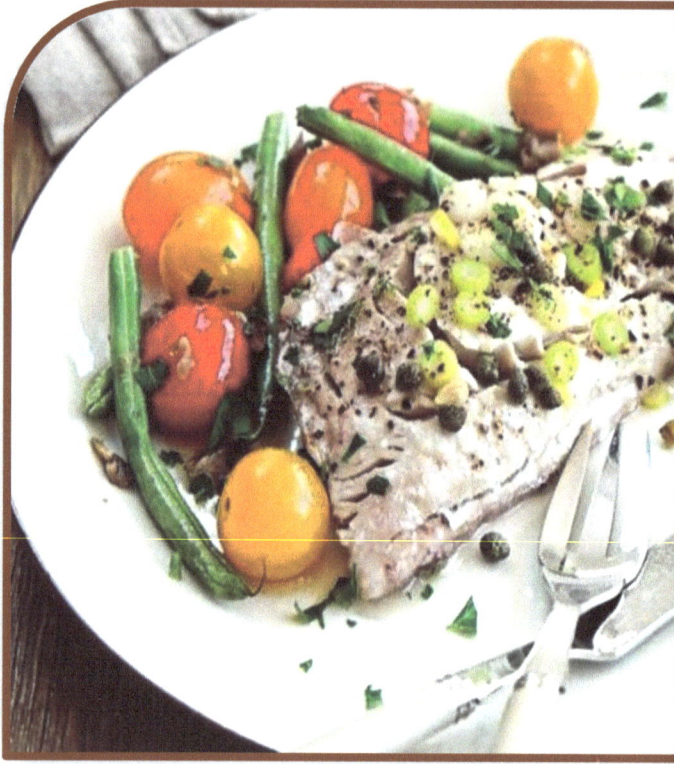

Ingredients

For the tomatoes
- 375g/13oz mixed red and yellow cherry tomatoes
- 320g/11½oz fine green beans, trimmed
- 2 garlic cloves, finely chopped
- 2 tbsp lemon juice
- low-calorie cooking spray
- salt and freshly ground black pepper

For the red mullet
- 8 red mullet fillets, approximately 100g/3½oz each
- 1 lemon, finely grated rind only
- 2 tsp baby capers, drained
- 2 spring onions, finely sliced

To garnish
- 2 tbsp chopped parsley
- 8 caper berries

Directions:

1. Preheat the oven to 200C/180C Fan/Gas 6.
2. Put the tomatoes in an ovenproof dish with the beans, garlic, lemon juice and spray with the oil. Season with salt and freshly ground black pepper and mix well. Bake for 10 minutes, or until the tomatoes and beans are tender.
3. Meanwhile, tear off 4 large sheets of foil and line with non-stick baking paper. Place 2 fish fillets on each piece of baking paper, then scatter over the lemon rind, capers, and spring onions, season with salt and freshly ground black pepper. Fold over the paper-lined foil and scrunch the edges together to seal. Place the parcels on a large baking tray.
4. Place the fish parcels next to the vegetables in the oven and bake for a further 8-10 minutes, or until the flesh flakes easily when pressed in the center with a knife.
5. Spoon the vegetables on to four serving plates and top each with two fish fillets. Garnish with the parsley and caperberries and serve.

11. GARLIC MUSHROOM FRITTATA

Prep Time: less than 30 mins Cooking Time: 10-30 mins

Servings: 2

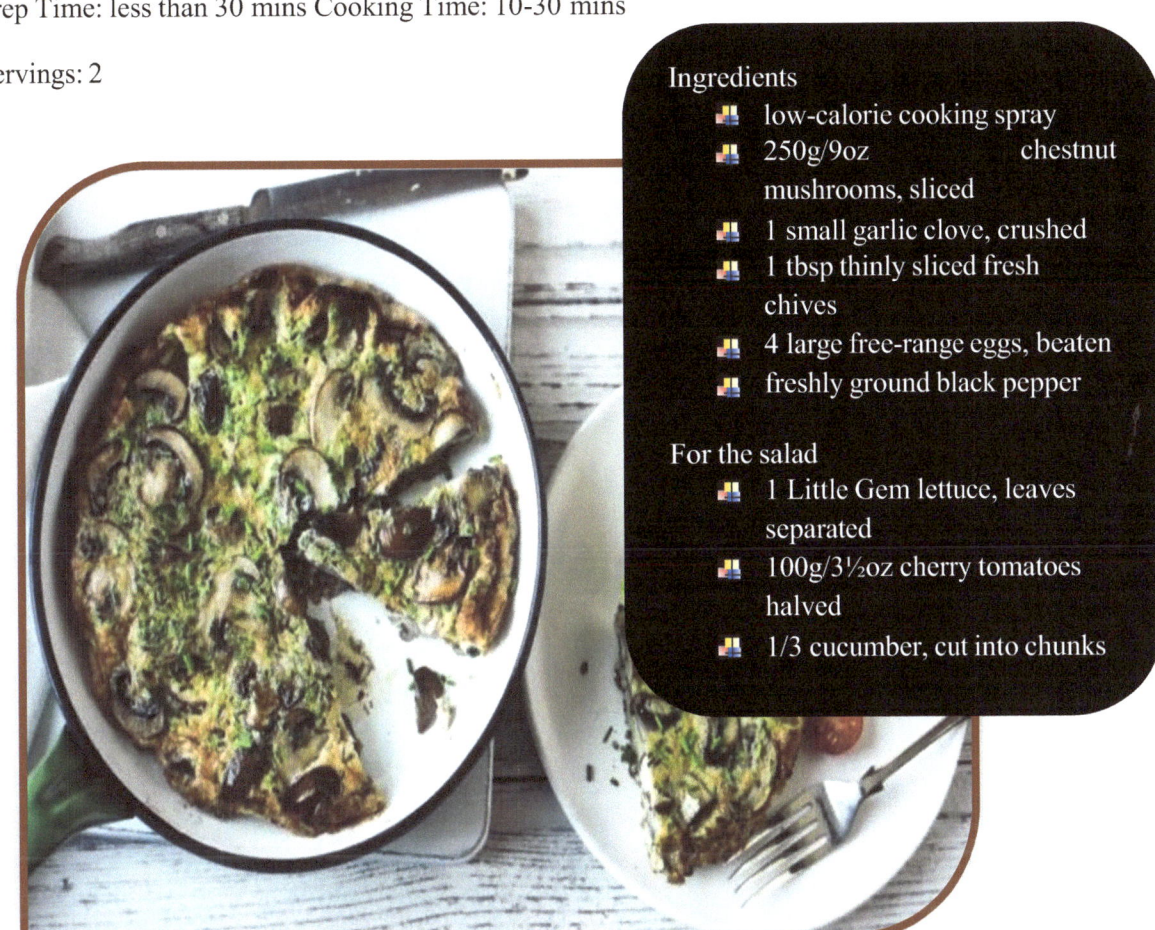

Ingredients
- low-calorie cooking spray
- 250g/9oz chestnut mushrooms, sliced
- 1 small garlic clove, crushed
- 1 tbsp thinly sliced fresh chives
- 4 large free-range eggs, beaten
- freshly ground black pepper

For the salad
- 1 Little Gem lettuce, leaves separated
- 100g/3½oz cherry tomatoes halved
- 1/3 cucumber, cut into chunks

Directions:
- Spray a small, flame-proof frying pan with oil and place over
- a high heat. (The base of the pan shouldn't be wider than about 18cm/7in.) Stir-fry the mushrooms in three batches for 2-3 minutes, or until softened and lightly browned. Tip the cooked mushrooms into a sieve over a bowl to catch any juices – you don't want the mushrooms to become soggy.
- Return all the mushrooms to the pan and stir in the garlic and chives, and a pinch of ground black pepper. Cook for a further minute, then reduces the heat to low.
- Preheat the grill to its hottest setting. Pour the eggs over the mushrooms. Cook for five minutes, or until almost set.
- Place the pan under the grill for 3-4 minutes, or until set.
- Combine the salad ingredients in a bowl.
- Remove from the grill and loosen the sides of the frittata with a round-bladed knife. Turn out onto a board and cut into wedges. Serve hot or cold with the salad.

12. BERRY YOGURT

Prep Time: less than 30 mins Cooking Time: 0 mins

Servings: 2

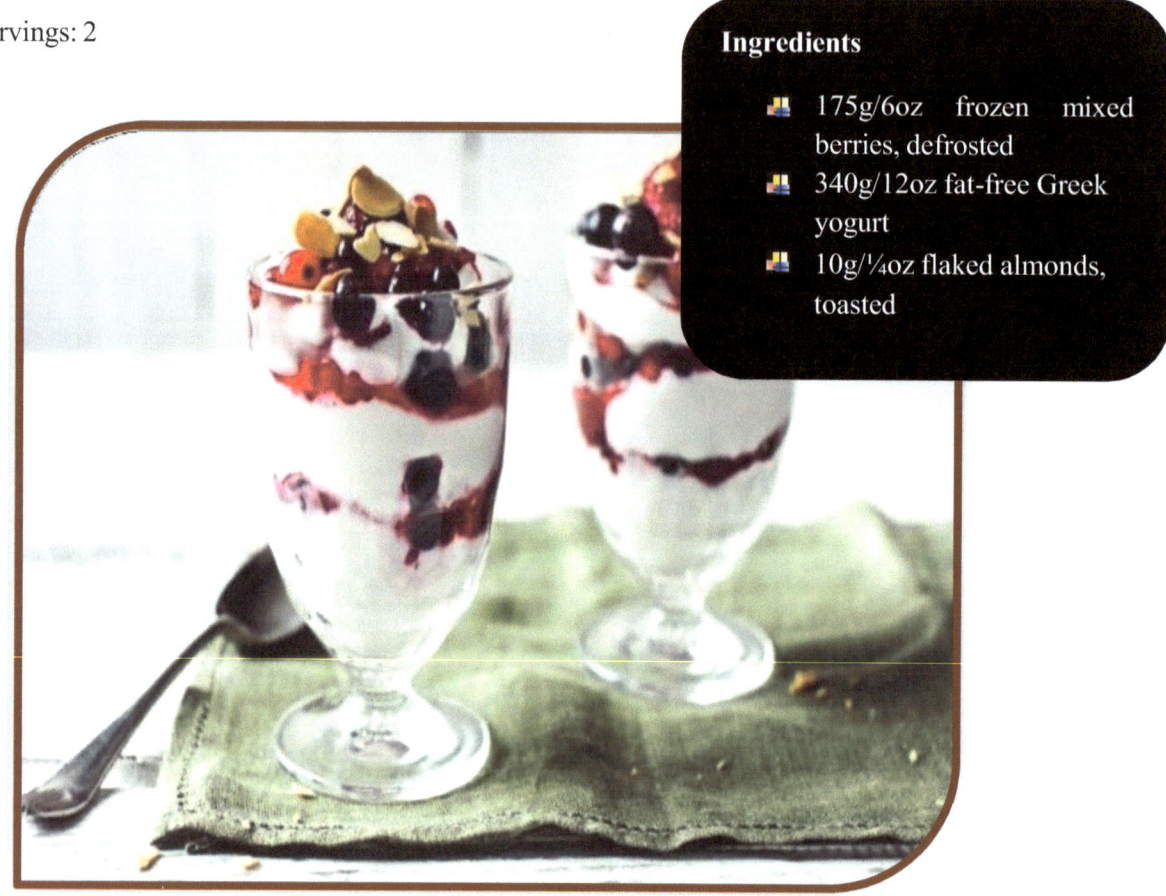

Ingredients

- 175g/6oz frozen mixed berries, defrosted
- 340g/12oz fat-free Greek yogurt
- 10g/¼oz flaked almonds, toasted

Directions:

1. Spoon the yogurt into two glasses, top with half the berries, and then repeat the layers.
2. Sprinkle with the flaked almonds and serve.

13. CAPONATA RATATOUILLE

Prep Time: less than 30 mins Cooking Time: 30 mins to 1 hour

Servings: 6

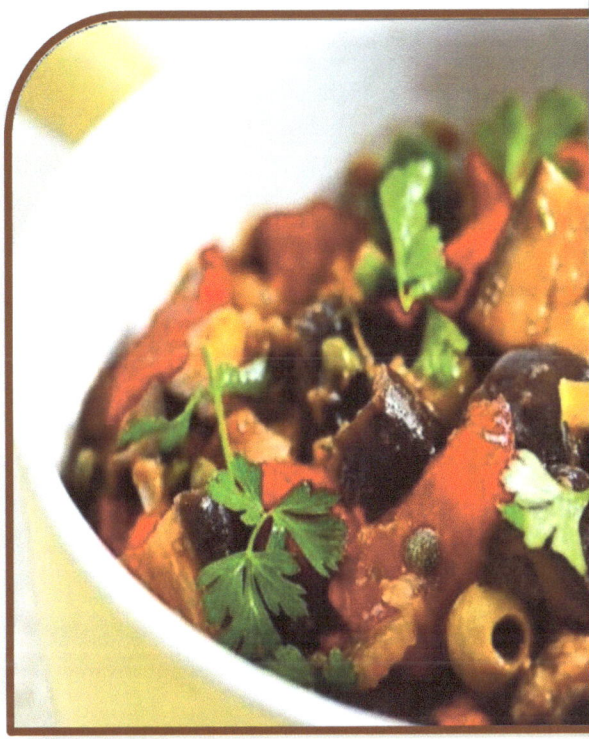

Ingredients
- 1 tbsp olive oil
- 750g/1lb 10oz aubergines, cut into 1cm/1½in chunks
- 1 large onion, cut into 1cm/1½in chunks
- 3 celery sticks, roughly chopped
- 2 large beef tomatoes, skinned and deseeded
- 1 tsp chopped thyme
- ¼-½ tsp cayenne pepper
- 2 tbsp capers, drained
- small handful pitted green olives
- 4 tbsp white wine vinegar
- 1 tbsp sugar
- 1-2 tbsp cocoa powder (optional)
- freshly ground black pepper

To garnish
- chopped almonds, toasted
- chopped parsley

Directions:

1. Heat the oil in a non-stick frying pan until very hot, add the aubergine and fry for about 15 minutes, or until very soft. Add a little boiling water to prevent sticking if necessary.
2. Meanwhile, place the onion and celery in a large saucepan with a little water. Cook for 5 minutes, or until tender but still firm.
3. Add the tomatoes, thyme, cayenne pepper and aubergine to the saucepan. Cook for 15 minutes, stirring occasionally. Add the capers, olives, vinegar, sugar and cocoa powder and cook for 2-3 minutes.
4. Season with freshly ground black pepper. Divide between 6 bowls, garnish with the toasted almonds and parsley and serve.

14. STIR-FRIED PORK WITH GINGER AND SOY SAUCE

Prep Time: less than 30 mins Cooking Time: 10-30 mins

Servings: 2

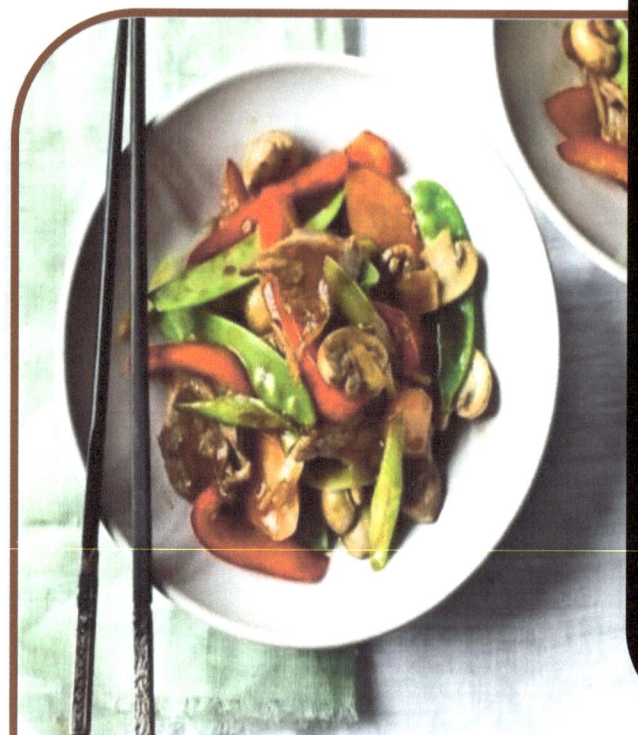

Ingredients

- 250g/9oz pork tenderloin, all visible fat removed, cut into chunks
- 1 tsp cornflour
- 2 tbsp dark soy sauce
- low-calorie cooking spray
- 150g/5½oz button mushrooms, sliced
- 2 red peppers, deseeded and sliced
- 75g/2½oz mangetout, trimmed
- 15g/½oz fresh root ginger, cut into thin matchsticks
- 1 garlic clove, thinly sliced
- 4 spring onions, cut into short lengths
- freshly ground black pepper

Directions:

1. Season the pork with pepper. Mix the cornflour with two tablespoons of cold water until smooth, then stir in the soy sauce.
2. Spray a large wok, or deep frying pan, with cooking spray and place over high heat. Stir-fry the pork for 1-2 minutes, or until lightly browned but not cooked through. Transfer to a plate.
3. Return the pan to the heat, reduce the heat a little and spray with more oil. Stir-fry the mushrooms and pepper for 2 minutes.
4. Add the mangetout and cook for a minute. Add the ginger, garlic and spring onions and stir-fry for a few seconds.
5. Return the pork to the pan and pour over the soy sauce mixture. Cook for 1-2 minutes, or until the sauce has thickened and the pork is cooked through. Serve immediately.

15. CHICKEN AND VEGETABLE BALTI

Prep Time: less than 30 mins Cooking Time: 30 mins to 1 hour

Servings: 2

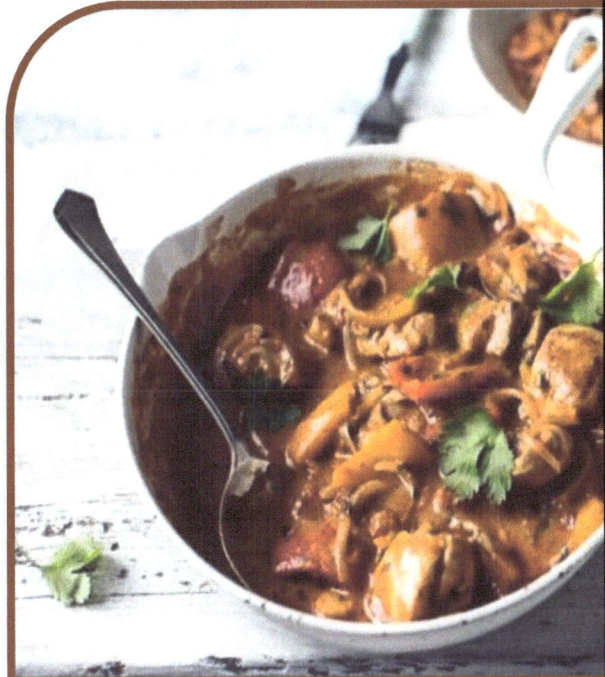

Ingredients
- calorie controlled cooking oil spray
- 1 medium onion, thinly sliced
- 4 chicken thighs, boned and skinned
- 1 red pepper, deseeded and cut into 3cm/1in chunks
- 1 yellow pepper, deseeded and cut into 3cm/1in chunks
- 1 tbsp cornflour
- 150g/5½oz fat-free natural yogurt
- 1 tbsp medium or mild curry powder
- 2 garlic cloves, thinly sliced
- 227g/8oz tin chopped tomatoes
- 3 heaped tbsp finely chopped fresh coriander, plus extra to garnish
- freshly ground black pepper

Directions:

1. Spray a large, deep, non-stick frying pan or wok with oil and place over medium heat. Add the onion and cook for five minutes, stirring regularly until well softened and lightly browned.
2. Meanwhile, trim all the visible fat off the chicken thighs, cut each one into four pieces and season with black pepper.
3. Add the chicken and peppers into the pan with the onion and cook for three minutes, turning occasionally.
4. Meanwhile, in a small bowl, mix the cornflour with 2 tablespoons cold water and stir in the yogurt until thoroughly mixed.
5. Sprinkle the curry powder over the chicken and vegetables, add the garlic and cook for 30 seconds.
6. Tip the tomatoes into the pan, add the yogurt mixture, 150ml/3½fl oz of water and coriander.
7. Bring to a gentle simmer and cook for 20-25 minutes, stirring occasionally until the chicken is tender and the sauce is thick.
8. Season with freshly ground black pepper to taste and garnish with coriander.

16. LAMB AND FLAGEOLET BEAN STEW

Prep Time: less than 30 mins Cooking Time: 1-2 hours

Servings: 4

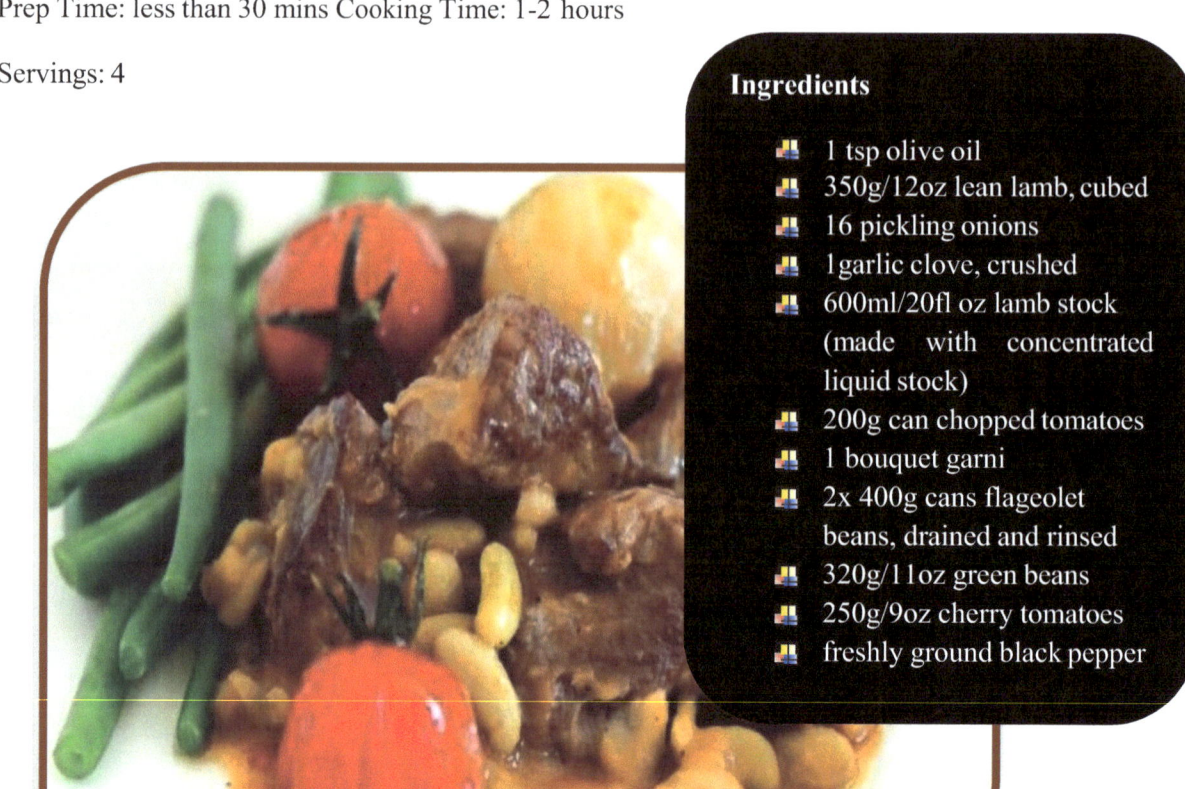

Ingredients

- 1 tsp olive oil
- 350g/12oz lean lamb, cubed
- 16 pickling onions
- 1 garlic clove, crushed
- 600ml/20fl oz lamb stock (made with concentrated liquid stock)
- 200g can chopped tomatoes
- 1 bouquet garni
- 2x 400g cans flageolet beans, drained and rinsed
- 320g/11oz green beans
- 250g/9oz cherry tomatoes
- freshly ground black pepper

Directions:

1. Heat the oil in a flameproof casserole or saucepan; add the lamb and fry for 3-4 minutes until browned all over. Remove the lamb from the casserole and set aside.
2. Add the onions and garlic to the pan and fry for 4-5 minutes, or until the onions are beginning to brown.
3. Return the lamb and any juices to the pan. Add the stock, tomatoes, bouquet garni and beans. Bring to the boil, stirring, then cover and simmer for 1 hour, or until the lamb is just tender.
4. Meanwhile, bring a pan of water to the boil and blanch the green beans. Place in a bowl of ice-cold water.
5. Add the cherry tomatoes to the stew and season well with freshly ground black pepper. Continue to simmer for 10 minutes.
6. Divide the stew between four plates, place the green beans alongside and serve.

17. KETO PORTOBELLO MUSHROOM MINI PIZZAS

Prep Time: 10 minutes Total Time: 20-25 minutes

Servings: 2

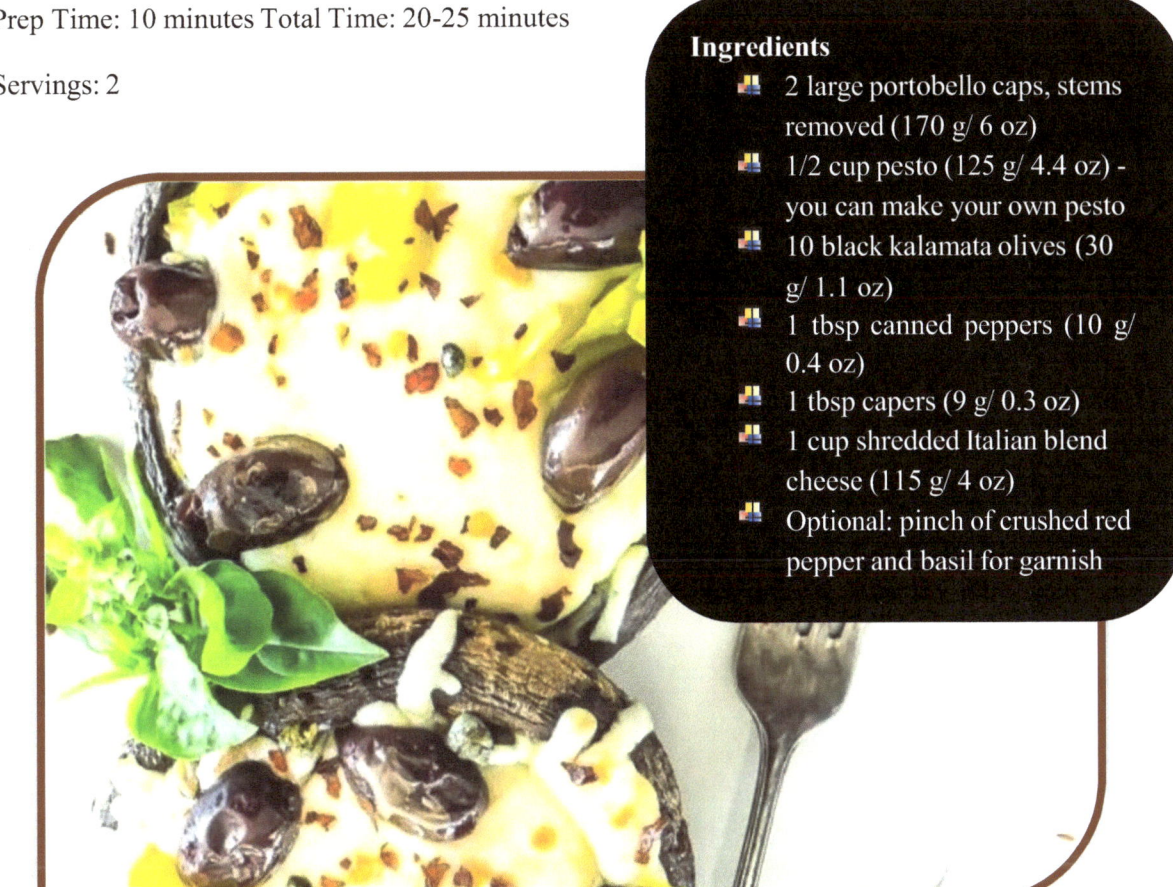

Ingredients
- 2 large portobello caps, stems removed (170 g/ 6 oz)
- 1/2 cup pesto (125 g/ 4.4 oz) - you can make your own pesto
- 10 black kalamata olives (30 g/ 1.1 oz)
- 1 tbsp canned peppers (10 g/ 0.4 oz)
- 1 tbsp capers (9 g/ 0.3 oz)
- 1 cup shredded Italian blend cheese (115 g/ 4 oz)
- Optional: pinch of crushed red pepper and basil for garnish

Directions:

1. Preheat oven to 190 °C/ 375 °F and place the mushrooms on a baking sheet. Divide the pesto between the mushrooms. (You can reserve the portobello stems and add them on top of your breakfast omelet.)
2. Tip for the perfect portobellos: Baked mushrooms can be watery. To reduce the moisture, brush the portobellos with a small amount of ghee or olive oil and bake without the topping for 10-12 minutes. Add the topping and broil on high for another 2-3 minutes.
3. Fill the centers with the cheese then top with your desired toppings.
4. Bake for 10-15 minutes, just until the cheese is bubbly and the mushrooms are starting to soften.
5. Serve immediately, optionally sprinkled with red pepper flakes, or refrigerate for up to a day and reheat before serving.

18. EASY PORK CHOPS WITH ASPARAGUS AND HOLLANDAISE

Prep Time: 10 minutes Total Time: 20-25 minutes

Servings: 3

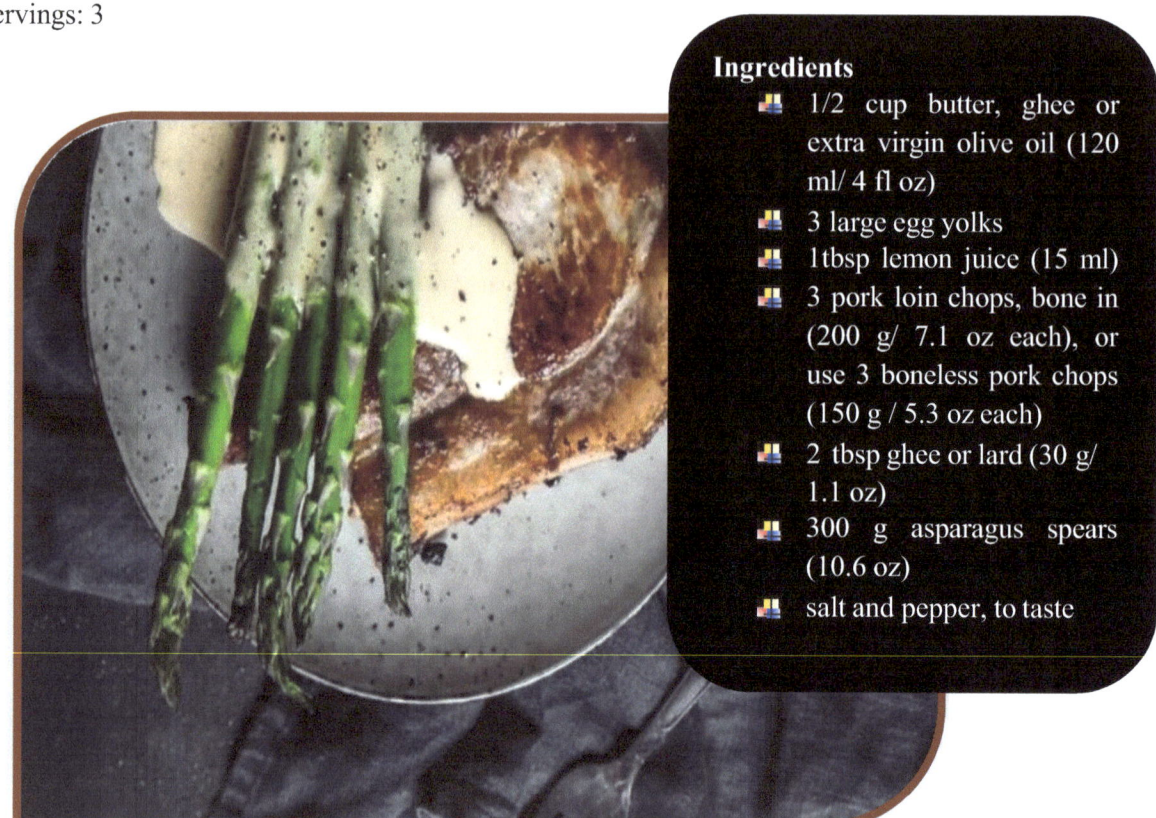

Ingredients
- 1/2 cup butter, ghee or extra virgin olive oil (120 ml/ 4 fl oz)
- 3 large egg yolks
- 1 tbsp lemon juice (15 ml)
- 3 pork loin chops, bone in (200 g/ 7.1 oz each), or use 3 boneless pork chops (150 g / 5.3 oz each)
- 2 tbsp ghee or lard (30 g/ 1.1 oz)
- 300 g asparagus spears (10.6 oz)
- salt and pepper, to taste

Directions:

1. Prepare the one-minute Hollandaise. Place 1/2 cup butter or ghee into a wide-mouthed jar, with enough room for a hand blender to fit into. Melt the butter in the microwave.
2. Add the egg yolks and the lemon juice. Place the hand blender in the bottom of the jar and blitz until well combined, lifting it slowly as you blend. Taste and season, if required.
3. Heat a frying pan over med-high heat and melt the remaining ghee. Cook the pork chops for 6 minutes on each side and then rest for 5 minutes.
4. Meanwhile, bring a pot of water to the boil and then blanch the asparagus for 5 minutes. Remove from the water and drain well.
5. Serve pork chops with asparagus spears placed over them, and then drizzle the hollandaise over the top.
6. Store the pork and asparagus in the refrigerator, wrapped for 2 days.
7. Store the hollandaise in its jar, with the lid on, in the refrigerator for 4 days, warming it before use.

19. LOW-CARB CHOCOLATE COCONUT SMOOTHIE

Prep Time: 5 minutes Total Time: 5 minutes

Servings: 1

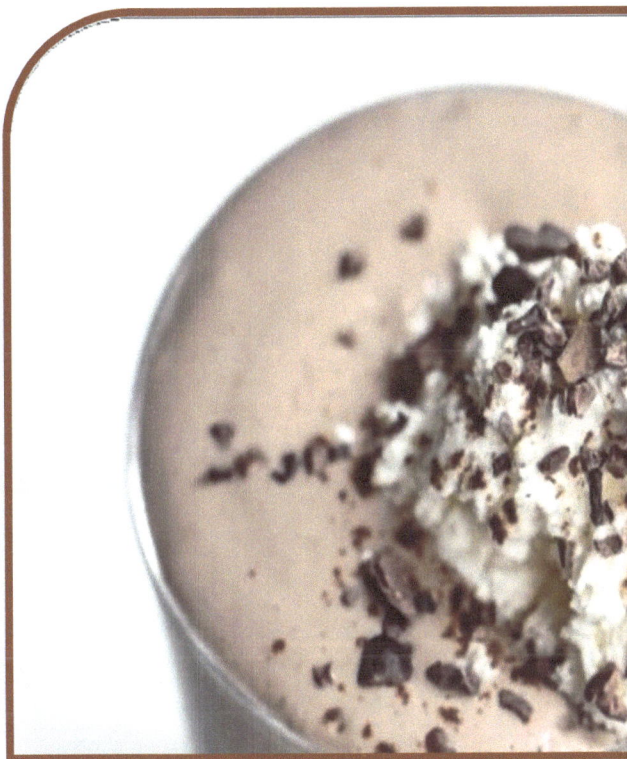

Ingredients
Smoothie:
- 1/2 large avocado (100 g/ 3.5 oz)
- 1 1/4 cup almond milk (300 ml/ 10 fl oz)
- 1/4 cup coconut cream or heavy whipping cream (60 ml/ 2 fl oz)
- 1 tbsp flax meal or chia seeds (7 g/ 0.3 oz)
- 1 1/2 tbsp cacao powder (8 g/ 0.3 oz)
- 1 tsp virgin coconut oil or MCT oil
- 1 heaped tbsp almond butter, or other nut or seed butter) (32 g/ 1.1 oz)
- Optional: water if too thick

Optional extras:
- 1-2 tbsp collagen for an extra protein boost
- healthy low-carb sweetener, to taste
- 1-2 tbsp whipped cream for topping
- 1 tsp cacao nibs or chopped dark chocolate for topping

Directions:

1. Place all the ingredients in a high-speed blender and blitz until smooth.
2. Pour the fat burning keto smoothie into a glass and serve. If using whipped cream for topping: Whip the coconut or heavy whipping cream using a hand blender until thick. Optionally, add cocoa nibs or chopped dark chocolate.
3. Best served fresh but can be stored in the fridge for 1 day.

20. ANTI KETO FLU NOURISH BOWL

Prep Time: 20 minutes Total Time: 20 minutes
Servings: 4

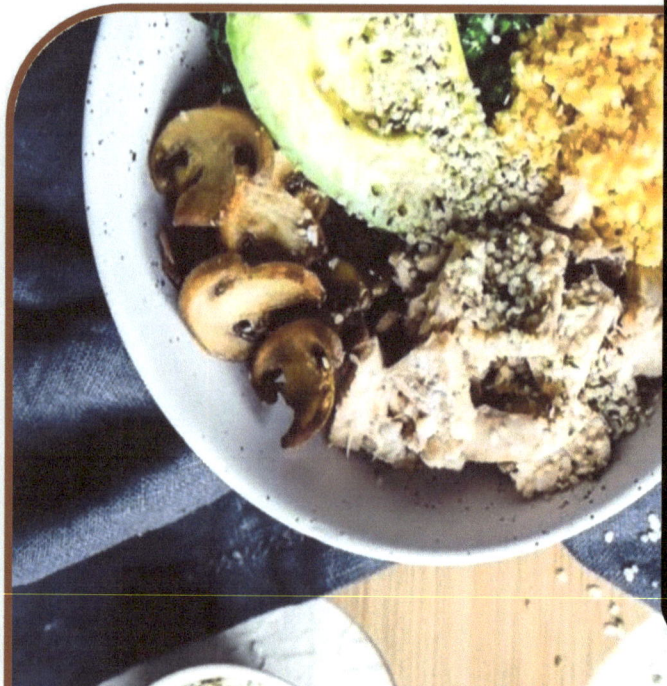

Ingredients
- 125 g lupin flakes (4.4 oz)
- 1 cup chicken broth or bone broth (240 ml/ 8 fl oz)
- 2 1/2 cups chopped dark-leaf kale or spinach (125 g/ 4.4 oz)
- 1 1/2 white mushrooms, sliced (105 g/ 3.7 oz)
- 1 can wild caught pink salmon, drained (150 g/ 5.3 oz)
- 1 tbsp ghee or virgin coconut oil (15 ml)
- 1/4 cup butter or ghee (60 g/ 2.1 oz)
- 1 clove garlic, minced
- 1/2 tsp sea salt, or to taste
- 1 large avocado, sliced (200 g/ 7.1 oz)
- 4 heaped tbsp hulled hemp seeds (60 g/ 2.1 oz)
- 2 tbsp extra virgin olive oil (30 ml)
- Optional: chile flakes, to taste

Directions:
1. Prepare all the ingredients. Clean and slice the mushrooms.
2. Place the lupin flakes into a microwaveable safe bowl and pour the chicken broth over. Stir through and set aside for 15 minutes.
3. Meanwhile, de-stem the kale and chop into small pieces. Finely mince the garlic.
4. Heat half of the ghee in a frying pan over high heat and sauté the kale, along with the garlic, until softened but still bright green. If you're using spinach, it will only take about 30 seconds to wilt.
5. Remove from pan and then cook mushrooms in the rest of the ghee in the pan. I like my mushrooms crispy on the outside and soft in the center, so I cook them well. Cook yours to your preferred doneness.
6. Drain salmon and check through for bones.
7. Once the lupin flakes have sat for 15 minutes, place them in the microwave for two minutes. Remove from the microwave and place pats of butter in to melt. Fluff up with a fork before serving.
8. Quarter your avocado and cut into slices.
9. Gather your ingredients and arrange them in your bowl in the way you like (recipe makes 4 bowls). Sprinkle with salt and dress with a good sprinkle of hemp seeds. Optionally, you can add a sprinkle of chili flakes for extra heat or a squeeze of lemon juice, if you would like some added zing.
10. Store in the refrigerator, without the avocado, covered for three days.

21. FAT HEAD PIZZA WITH MOZZARELLA, TOMATO & ROCKET

Prep Time: 10 minutes Total Time: 20-25 minutes

Servings: 4

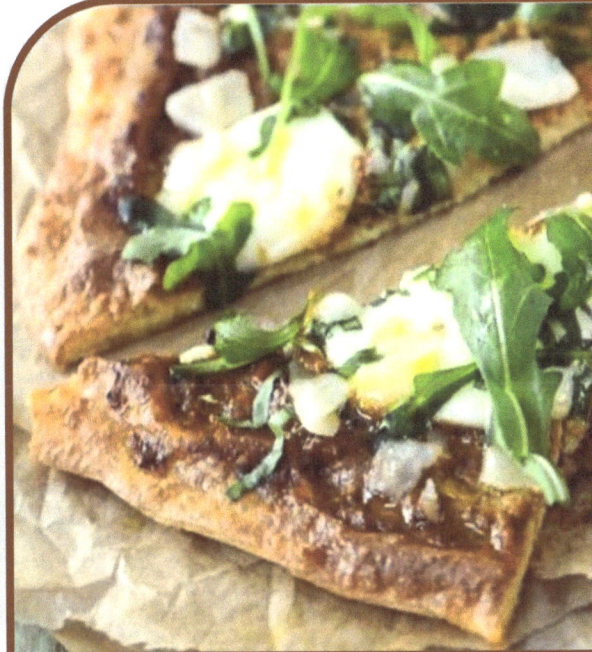

Ingredients

Fat Head Pizza Base:
- 1 1/2 cups grated mozzarella cheese (170 g/ 6 oz)
- 2 tbsp cream cheese (56 g/ 2 oz)
- 1 large egg
- 1/2 tsp salt
- 3/4 cup + 1 tbsp almond flour (85 g/ 3 oz)
- extra virgin olive oil for flattening the dough

Topping:
- 1/3 cup sugar-free Marinara sauce (80 g/ 2.8 oz)
- 4 1/2 oz fresh mozzarella cheese, sliced (125 g)
- fresh basil
- 1 cup fresh rocket (arugula)
- 1oz flaked Parmesan cheese (28 g)
- 2 tbsp extra virgin olive oil

Directions:

1. Start by making the pizza crust. Place the grated mozzarella cheese into a bowl and add the cream cheese. Microwave on high for 1 minute. Mix with a spatula and microwave on high for another 30 seconds. Mix again.
2. Add the egg and combine well. Add salt, almond flour, and mix until well combined.
3. Place the dough on a heatproof baking mat and use your hands to flatten ... until 1/4 - 1/2 inch (1/2 - 1 cm) thick. Spray some olive oil on your hands to prevent the dough from sticking.
4. Alternatively, you can use a piece of parchment paper on top and roll the dough out until thin. Dock the dough with a fork and bake in the oven preheated to 220 °C/ 425 °F for 12-15 minutes.
5. Remove from the oven and spread the marinara sauce on top. Add fresh mozzarella slices.
6. Place back in the oven for 5 minutes. Remove from the oven, top with fresh basil, rocket, Parmesan cheese, and drizzle with extra virgin olive oil. Fat Head Pizza with Mozzarella, Tomato & Rocket
7. Slice and serve hot or cold.
8. Enjoy!

22. LOW-CARB PHILLY CHEESE STEAK SALAD

Prep Time: 15 minutes Total Time: 30 minutes

Servings: 2

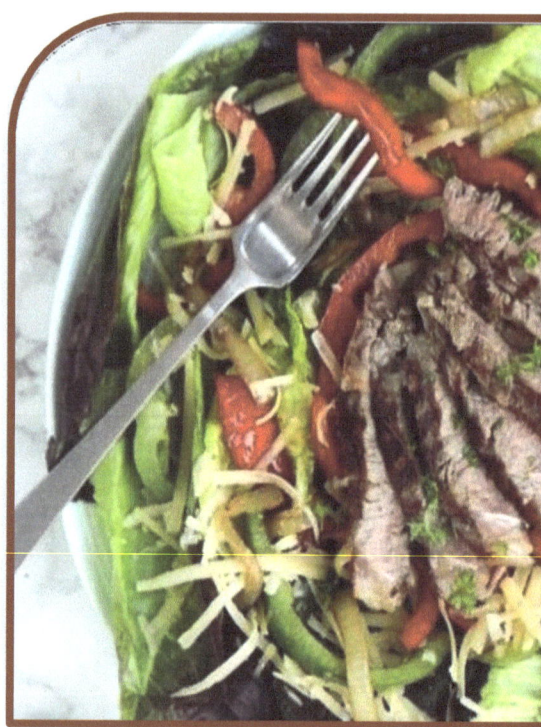

Ingredients

Steaks:
- 2 small or 1 large ribeye steak (300 g / 10.6 oz) - you could also use flank or skirt steak - make sure you cut it thinly after cooking
- 1/4 salt (I like pink Himalayan)
- freshly ground black pepper
- 1 tbsp ghee, lard or duck fat for greasing

Salad:
- 1 tbsp ghee, lard or duck fat
- 1 small white or yellow onion, sliced (70 g/ 2.5 oz)
- 1 clove garlic, minced
- 1 medium green pepper, sliced (120 g/ 4.2 oz)
- 1 medium red bell pepper, sliced (120 g/ 4.2 oz)
- 1/2 cup grated cheddar or provolone or mozzarella or any cheese you like (56 g/ 2 oz)
- 1 bag lettuce of mixed greens of choice (200 g/ 7.1 oz)
- salt, pepper and fresh herbs of choice for garnish.

Directions:

1. Allow the steak to sit at room temperature for 10-15 minutes.
2. Using a paper towel, pat the excess blood off. Toss with some of the melted ghee and season with salt and pepper. The ghee may solidify even at room temperature which is perfectly normal. Make sure you season the steak after you toss it with oil. You don't want to wash the seasoning off.
3. Fry in a very hot heavy based pan over high heat for 2-4 minutes on each side to seal in the juices. When you see the sides getting brown, it's time to flip it over. The exact time depends on the size of your steak. Small would take 2 minutes, while large up to 4 minutes to brown. Reduce to medium heat and continue to cook for further 4 minutes (rare), 7 minutes (medium), 11 minutes (well done). There is no need to turn the steak again. If you use a thermometer, the steak should read 52-60 °C/ 125-140 °F (rare to medium-rare).
4. You can use a cast iron griddle pan which is perfect for steaks.

5. Remove the steak from the pan and allow it to rest in a warm place for 5-7 minutes. The steak will finish cooking in the residual heat as the temperature slowly goes down. The best way to rest the steak is to fold it up in a parchment paper and then in a kitchen towel. This will keep it juicy and equally pink inside.
6. After 5-7 minutes, slice into thin strips.
7. While the steak is resting, prepare the vegetables. Add a tablespoon of ghee to the pan where you cooked the steak. Place the sliced onion, minced garlic, green pepper and red pepper in the pan and cook over medium-high heat for 3-5 minutes, until crisp-tender. Do not overcook the vegetables.
8. Assemble the salad. Place the lettuce, warm peppers and onion, grated cheddar cheese and thinly cut steak into a serving bowl. If you like the cheese to be melted, add it on top of the warm vegetables together with sliced steak while still in the hot pan and let it melt - then transfer to the bowl on top of lettuce.
9. Serve immediately while still warm.

23. KETO CALIFORNIA EGGS BENEDICT

Prep Time: 20 minutes Total Time: 20 minutes

Servings: 2

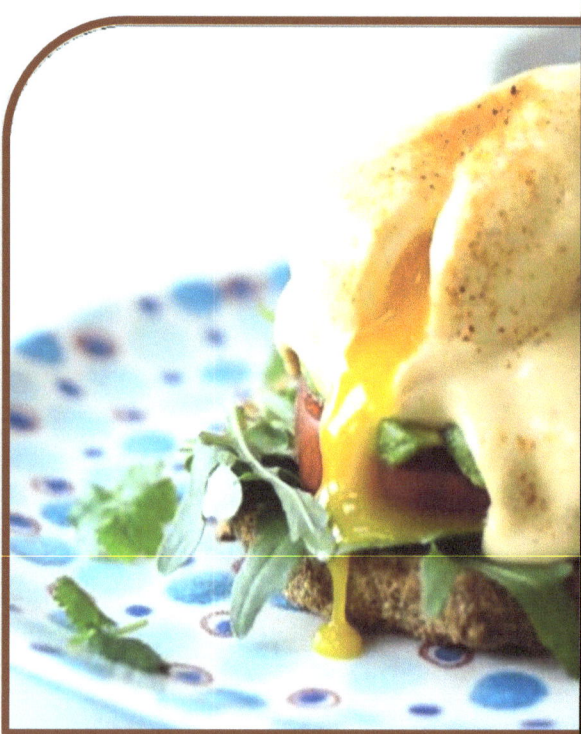

Ingredients
Eggs Benedict:
- 1 keto bun, halved (you can use Ultimate Keto Bun or Nut-Free Keto Bun) - will take an extra hour to prepare
- a handful of fresh greens such as arugula (rocket) (20 g/ 0.7 oz)
- 2 large slices of tomato (60 g/ 2.1 oz)
- 1/2 medium avocado, sliced (75 g/ 2.7 oz)
- 2 large eggs, poached
- pinch of paprika or cayenne pepper

Spicy Hollandaise Sauce:
- 2 large egg yolks
- 1/2 tsp Dijon mustard (you can make your own)
- 2 tbsp fresh lemon juice or lime juice (30 ml)
- 1/4 cup extra virgin olive oil (60 ml/ 2 fl oz)
- 1-2 tbsp water if too thick
- 1 tbsp Sriracha sauce (you can make your own)
- salt and pepper to taste

Directions:

1. Cut the keto bun in half. Optionally, place under a broiler for a few minutes to crisp up.
2. Poach the eggs. Fill a saucepan with water and add a dash of white vinegar and a pinch of salt. Crack the egg into a cup. Once the water is boiling, reduce the heat to low. Create a gentle whirlpool in the water to help the egg white wrap around the yolk.
3. Slowly tip the egg in the center of the whirlpool, lowering the cup an inch into the water. Cook undisturbed for 3 minutes. Remove the egg from the hot water and place in a bowl with cold water for a few seconds. This will prevent the egg from overcooking. Then transfer the egg to a plate and keep warm.
4. Prepare the Hollandaise sauce. In a bowl, mix the egg yolks, Dijon mustard, and lemon juice. Fill a medium saucepan with about a cup of water and bring to a boil over a medium heat.

5. Place the bowl with the egg yolk mixture over the saucepan and make sure the water doesn't touch the bottom of the bowl. Keep mixing until the egg yolk mixture starts to thicken.
6. Slowly pour the olive oil into the mixture until thick and creamy. Keep stirring at all times to avoid clumping. If the Hollandaise is too thick, add a splash of water. If it clumps, place in a blender and pulse until smooth.
7. Finally, take off the heat and add the Sriracha sauce, salt, and pepper. Set aside and keep warm. Keto California Eggs Benedict
8. To assemble the Eggs Benedict, place a slice of keto bun on 2 plates. Top each one with leafy greens, a slice of tomato and sliced avocado.
9. Top each one with poached egg and pour over the Hollandaise sauce. Garnish with a pinch of paprika or cayenne pepper. Serve immediately.

24. LOW-CARB BEEF STEW WITH HERBY DUMPLINGS

Prep Time: 40 minutes Total Time: 3 hours 15 minutes

Servings: 6

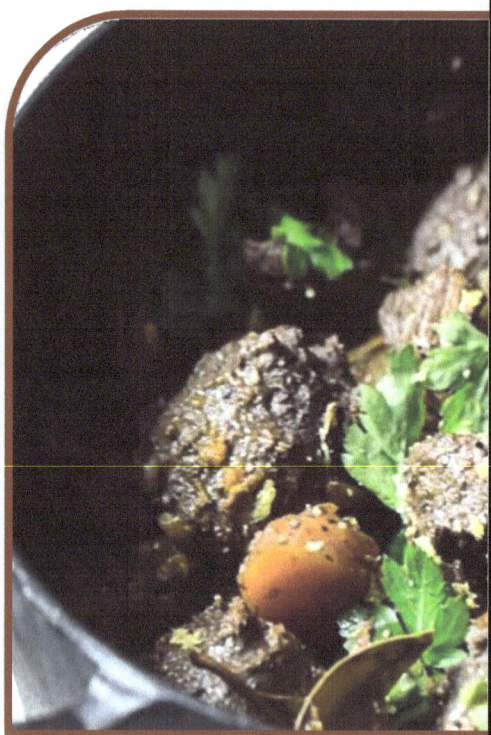

Ingredients

Stew:
- 900 g stewing beef such as braising steak (2 lb)
- 2 tbsp extra virgin olive oil or ghee
- 1 medium red onion, chopped (100 g/ 3.5 oz)
- 200 g pumpkin, ideally Hokkaido (7.1 oz)
- 1 medium carrot (60 g/ 2.1 oz)
- 3 bay leaves
- 3 sprigs of fresh rosemary
- 2 cloves garlic, minced
- 2 tbsp tomato puree (30 g/ 1.1 oz)
- 1/2 cup dry red wine (120 ml/ 4 fl oz)
- 2 cups beef stock or beef bone broth (480 ml/ 16 fl oz) - you can make your own
- 3/4 tsp sea salt or pink Himalayan salt, or to taste
- 1/4 tsp cracked black pepper

Dumplings (makes 12):
- 3 large egg whites
- 1 large egg
- 1 cup water, boiling (240 ml/ 8 fl oz)
- 3/4 cup almond flour (75 g/ oz)
- 1/3 cup sesame seed flour (30 g/ 1.1 oz)
- 1/4 cup coconut flour (30 g/ 1.1 oz)
- 2 1/2 tbsp psyllium husk powder (20 g/ oz)
- 1 1/2 tsp gluten-free baking powder
- 1/4 tsp pink Himalayan or sea salt
- 1 tbsp chopped rosemary
- 1 tbsp fresh thyme

To serve:
- 1 tsp fresh lemon zest (about 1/2 lemon)
- pinch cracked black pepper
- fresh parsley for topping

Directions:

1. Preheat the oven to 160 °C/ 320 °F (fan assisted). Heat 1 tablespoon of olive oil in a large pan. Brown the meat on medium heat for 5 minutes, stirring regularly to seal the meat for approximately 5 minutes. Turn off the heat and place to one side.
2. Meanwhile, peel the onion, pumpkin, and carrots and chop into chunks about 2 cm (1 inch). In another pan heat one tablespoon of

olive oil and fry the vegetables on medium heat for 10 minutes, stirring regularly to prevent sticking.
3. Add the beef, rosemary, bay leaves, chopped garlic, and tomato puree. Sauté for a further 2 minutes.
4. Add the red wine, reduce the heat and simmer for 5 minutes.
5. Add the stock, season with salt and pepper, bring to the boil.
6. Place a casserole dish in the oven to heat up. Place the stew in the casserole dish and add a lid. Roast in the oven for 3 hours until the meat is tender and the juices have concentrated. Remove from the oven once cooked. Turn up the oven to 175 °C/ 350 °F.
7. Make the dumplings as per the keto bread recipe 1. Grease a cupcake tin with olive oil to prevent sticking. Shape into dumpling shapes (3 to 4 cm/ up to 1-1/2 inch in diameter) and place individually in the cupcake holes. Bake in the oven for 25 minutes. Turn over with a spoon and place back in the oven to cook for a further 5 minutes.
8. Place the stew back in the oven to heat through if cooled slightly. Add the dumplings.
9. To serve, place the stew in bowls and top with grated lemon zest, fresh parsley and a pinch of cracked black pepper.

25. THE BEST KETO CHEESEBURGER

Prep Time: 20 minutes Total Time: 20 minutes

Servings: 4

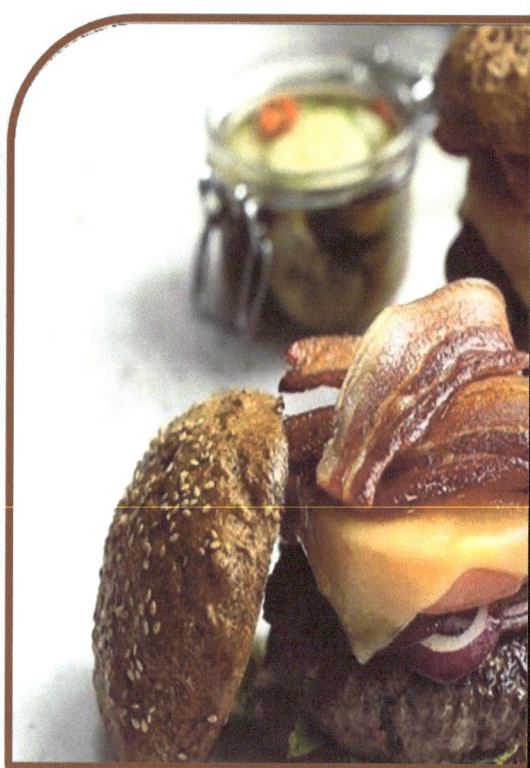

Ingredients
Burger Patties:
- 600 g ground beef (1.3 lb)
- 1 clove garlic, minced
- 2 tsp onion powder
- 1 tsp apple cider vinegar
- 1 tsp sea salt
- 1 tsp black pepper
- 1tbsp ghee or lard for greasing (15 ml)

Burger sauce:
- 1/4 cup paleo mayonnaise (55 g/ 1.9 oz) - you can make your own mayo
- 2tbsp sugar-free ketchup or tomato puree (30 g/ 1.1 oz) - you can make your own ketchup
- 1 tbsp pickle juice or lemon juice (15 ml)
- salt and pepper, to taste

Burgers:
- 4 Ultimate Keto Buns or Nut-Free Keto Buns
- 2 tbsp butter, melted (30 ml)
- 4 slices slices bacon, cut lenghtwise (120 g/ 4.2 oz)
- 2 cups green shredded lettuce (60 g/ 2.1 oz)
- 16 slices sugar-free pickles (40 g/ 1.4 oz) - you can make your own pickles
- 8 slices red onion (60 g/ 2.1 oz)
- 4 slices tomato, sliced (120 g/ 4.2 oz)
- 4 slices slices cheddar, provolone or Monterey Jack cheese (85 g/ 3 oz)

Directions:

1. Prepare the keto burger buns. If you don't have any, you'll need an extra hour to prepare them.
2. I brushed a batch of these buns with one egg yolk mixed with a tablespoon of water which gave them a shiny finish. You can make any keto bread in advance, freeze and defrost at room temperature.
3. In a bowl, mix the ingredients for the burger patties: beef, minced garlic, onion powder, apple cider vinegar, sea

salt, and black pepper. Do not overmix or the burgers will become tough.
4. Using your hands, create 4 equal patties, 1/2 to 3/4 inch (1 1/4 to 2 cm) thick. Use your hands to smooth any cracks.
5. Pierce the patties with a fork several times. This will loosen the patties and help them cook equally without curling or getting tough while enabling maximum caramelization. Set aside.
6. Prepare the burger sauce by mixing the mayonnaise, ketchup, pickle juice, salt, and pepper. Set aside.
7. To brown the keto burger buns, cut them widthwise. Brush them with melted butter and cook in a hot skillet cut side down for about a minute or until browned and crispy. Remove from the skillet and set aside.
8. Grease the hot skillet with a tablespoon of ghee and add the burger patties. The patties should sizzle as soon as they touch the skillet. Do not crowd the pan - work in batches. Cook over high heat, until a crust forms on the bottom and the burgers, are easy to flip on the other side. This will take 2-3 minutes.
9. Once flipped, cook until the crust forms on the bottom and the sides are browned. Do not pierce the burgers with a fork or you will lose the juices. It will take another 2-3 minutes to cook through. The thicker the patties, the longer they will take to cook. Transfer to a plate and set aside.
10. In the same pan, cook the bacon slices. Cut each of the slices lengthwise and cook until browned and crispy. Alternatively, bake in the oven.
11. To assemble the burger: Spread about 2 teaspoons of the burger sauce on each bun halve. Top each the bottom half with 4 slices of pickles and add a quarter of the shredded lettuce.
12. Add a burger patty, 2 onion slices, 1 slice of tomato and 1 slice of cheese.
13. Place under a broiler for a minute until the cheese is melted.
14. Otherwise, you can add the cheese directly on top of the burger patty while still hot (see more in step 8). Finally, top with 2 slices of cooked bacon and add the top half of the burger bun.
15. Enjoy! Serve with leftover burger sauce, or low-carb ketchup and homemade Dijon mustard. Optionally, serve with more pickles or a big bowl of crispy vegetable salad drizzled with olive oil and lemon juice.

26. HEALTHY SESAME CRUSTED SALMON WITH COCONUT CAULI-RICE

Prep Time: 10 minutes Total Time: 25 minutes

Servings: 2

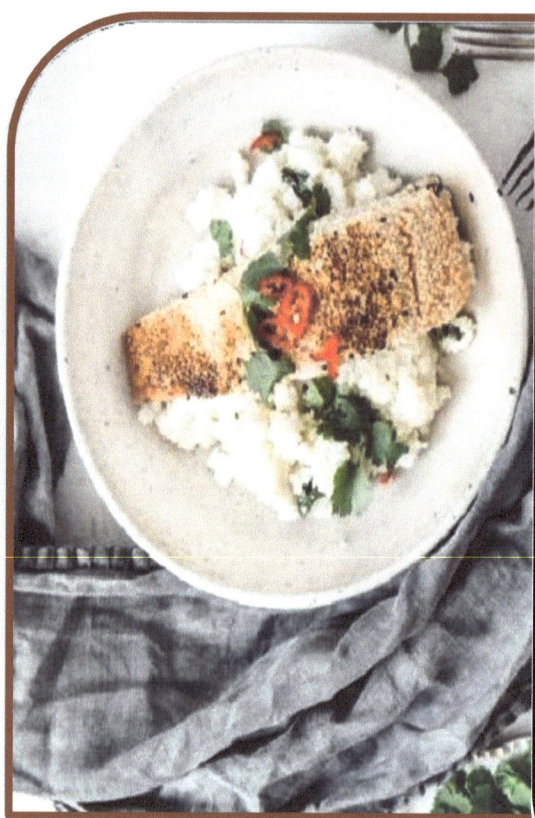

Ingredients

Sesame-crusted salmon:
- 2 large wild salmon fillets (400 g/ 14.1 oz)
- 1/4 cup sesame seeds (36 g/ 1.3 oz)
- 2 tbsp virgin coconut oil (30 ml)

Coconut cauliflower rice:
- 1/2 medium cauliflower (300 g/ 10.6 oz)
- 2 tbsp virgin coconut oil (30 ml)
- 1/2 tsp sea salt
- 1 tsp Erythritol or Swerve
- 1/3 cup coconut cream (80 ml)
- 1/4 cup fresh cilantro (coriander) leaves, plus more to serve
- Optional: 1 small red chili, thinly sliced

Directions:

1. Place cauliflower in a food processor and process until it resembles rice, being careful not to over process. Cutting the cauliflower into smaller florets, or using a grating blade, will help with this.
2. Heat a pan over medium heat. Add the coconut oil, and once hot, add the cauliflower. Cook, stirring, for around five minutes until the cauliflower is nearly cooked through. Add the salt, Erythritol and stir to combine, and then add the coconut cream.
3. Cook, stirring, another minute or so until the coconut cream is absorbed. Stir through coriander and chili and set aside.
4. Heat another pan over medium heat. Place the sesame seeds on a plate or shallow bowl, and coat both fillets with the seeds.
5. Once the pan is hot, add the remaining 2 tablespoons of coconut oil, and gentle place in the salmon fillets.
6. Cook 6 – 8 minutes, turning halfway through. Note that for really thick fillets, you may need an extra minute or two.

27. EASY AVOCADO & BACON SALAD

Prep Time: 10 minutes Total Time: 20 minutes

Servings: 2

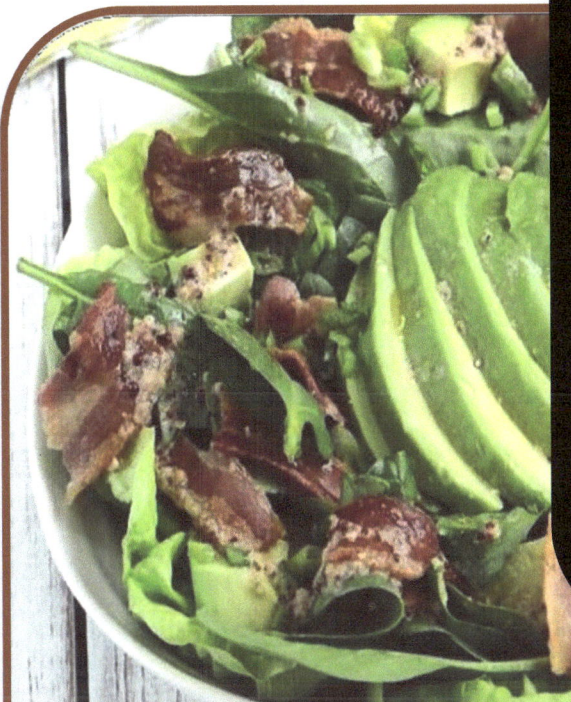

Ingredients
- 2 large avocados (400 g / 14.2 oz)
- 2 small heads lettuce (200 g / 7.1 oz)
- 2 cups fresh spinach (60 g / 2.1 oz)
- 1 medium spring onion (15 g / 0.5 oz)
- 4 large slices bacon, outdoor-reared (120 g / 4.2 oz)
- Optionally: 2 hard-boiled eggs, sliced

Vinaigrette:
- 3 tbsp extra virgin olive oil
- 1 tbsp apple cider vinegar or home-made fruit vinegar
- 1 tsp Dijon mustard or whole grain mustard (make your own)
- pinch salt (I like pink Himalayan)
- freshly ground black pepper
- Optionally: dash Tabasco

Directions:

1. Start by crisping up the bacon. Place the slices in a hot pan.
2. Add 1/2 cup of water and cook over medium heat to render the fat and until the bacon is crisped up, for 10-15 minutes. When done, set aside.
3. Meanwhile, tear the lettuce and wash well with the spinach.
4. Place in a salad spinner or pat dry with a kitchen towel. Halve and deseed the avocados and slice into stripes.
5. Make the vinaigrette by mixing all the ingredients.
6. Optionally, peel and slice the hard-boiled eggs.
7. To cook the eggs: Fill a small saucepan with water up to three quarters. Add a good pinch of salt. This will prevent the eggs from cracking. Bring to a boil. Using a spoon or hand, dip each egg in and out of the boiling water (be careful not to get burnt!). This will prevent the egg from cracking, as the temperature change won't be so dramatic. To get the eggs hard-boiled, you need around 10 minutes. When done, remove from the heat and place in a bowl filled with cold water.
8. Assemble the salad by folding the lettuce and spinach in a bowl, add crisped up bacon torn in smaller pieces and sliced avocado. Enjoy!

28. KETO CHICKEN PIE

Prep Time: 30 minutes Total time: 60 minutes

Servings: 8

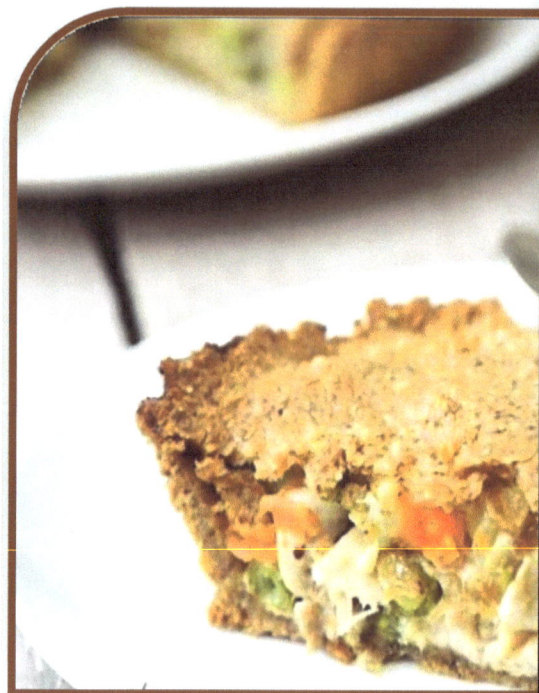

Ingredients

Crust (1 1/2 recipe Savory Keto Pie Crust) - this means you'll need:
- 3 cups pork rinds, powdered (150 g / 5.3 oz) - you can make your own
- 1 1/2 cup almond flour (150 g / 5.3 oz)
- 1/4 cup + 3 tbsp flax meal (60 g / 2.1 oz)
- 3 large eggs, free-range or organic
- 1/2 tsp salt if using unsalted pork rinds

Filling:
- 5 chicken thighs (500 g / 17.6 oz / 1.1 lb)
- 1 cup green beans (200 g / 7.1 oz)
- 1 medium carrot (70 g / 2.5 oz)
- 1/2 medium celeriac (130 g / 4.6 oz)
- 1 large onion (150 g / 5.3 oz)
- 1/2 cup butter or ghee - you can make your own (110 g / 4 oz)
- 1/2 cup heavy whipping cream (120 ml / 4 fl oz)
- 1-quart water or chicken stock, enough to cover the chicken and vegetables (1 l)
- 2 tbsp freshly chopped parsley

Directions:

1. Prepare the Savory Keto Crust by following this recipe. - just make 1 1/2 the amount of the recipe to have enough crust for the top of the pie. Only use 2/3 of the dough to press in the pan - leave the rest for the top of the pie and keep it in the fridge.
2. Bake for 12-15 minutes (see detailed instructions here). When the pie crust is done, remove from the oven and let it cool down.
3. When cooled, loosen the crust from the edges and bottom - use a sharp knife if needed.
4. Meanwhile, dice the chicken thighs, peel and slice the carrot.
5. Peel and dice the celeriac and cut the green beans into thirds.
6. Place everything into a saucepan and add the water and salt.
7. Bring to a boil, then reduce to medium-low, cover with a lid and cook for 15-20 minutes. Keto Chicken Pie

7. Divide the cauliflower rice between two plates, and then place a cooked salmon fillet on top of each. Top with extra coriander leaves, and serve immediately.

8. Meanwhile, peel and finely chop the onion. Place on a pan with all of the butter (or ghee) and cook over medium heat until caramelized. This can take up to 15 minutes - mix to prevent burning.
9. Preheat the oven to 200 °C/ 400 °F. When the chicken & vegetables are cooked, pour the stock through a sieve and keep the vegetables and meat in the pot - set aside.
10. Pour the cream into the pan with the onion and stir to combine well. Add 1/4 cup - 3/4 cup of the chicken & vegetable stock and mix well. When done, season with salt and set aside. Keep the remaining stock for another recipe.
11. Roll out the remaining dough for the top of the pie. You'll need to place the dough between two pieces of parchment paper while rolling to avoid tearing the dough. Try to achieve a round shape that will fit the pie.
12. Place the drained chicken & vegetables into the pie crust. Add freshly chopped parsley and pour in the creamed onion and spread evenly over the topping.
13. Top with the remaining rolled out dough and press towards the edges.
14. Using a knife, make several small slits in the top to allow steam to escape. Place in the oven and bake for about 30 minutes.
15. When done, remove from the oven and set aside for 10-15 minutes before serving. Enjoy!

29. CHICKEN CLUB LETTUCE WRAP SANDWICH

Prep Time: 5 mins Cook Time: 5 mins Total Time: 10 mins

Servings: 1

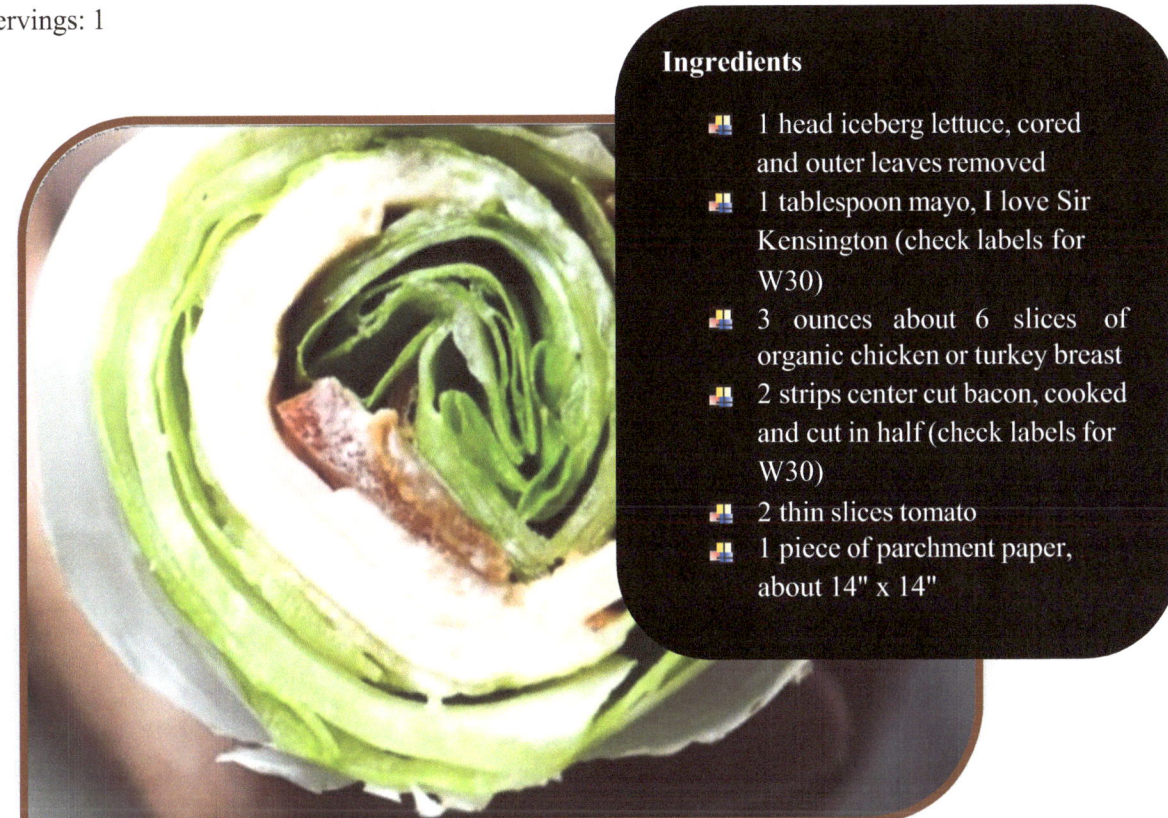

Ingredients

- 1 head iceberg lettuce, cored and outer leaves removed
- 1 tablespoon mayo, I love Sir Kensington (check labels for W30)
- 3 ounces about 6 slices of organic chicken or turkey breast
- 2 strips center cut bacon, cooked and cut in half (check labels for W30)
- 2 thin slices tomato
- 1 piece of parchment paper, about 14" x 14"

Directions:

1. Place the parchment paper down on your work surface.
2. Layer 6 to 7 large leaves of lettuce in the middle of parchment paper so that you create a lettuce base about 9 inches by 10 inches.
3. Spread the mayo in the center of the lettuce wrap.
4. Layer with the chicken or turkey, bacon and tomato.
5. Starting with the end closest to you, roll the lettuce wraps jelly roll style using the parchment as your base as tight as possible.
6. Halfway through rolling, tuck the ends of the wraps towards the middle.
7. Continue to roll the lettuce wrap, keeping it as tight as possible and using the parchment paper to guide you.
8. When it is completely wrapped, roll the remainder of the parchment around the lettuce tightly.
9. Using a serrated knife, cut the lettuce wrap almost completely, leaving a small piece of the parchment intact to help hold it together.

30. QUICK & EASY CHICKEN SPRING ROLL

Prep Time 15 mins Cook Time 15 mins Total Time 30 mins

Servings: 4

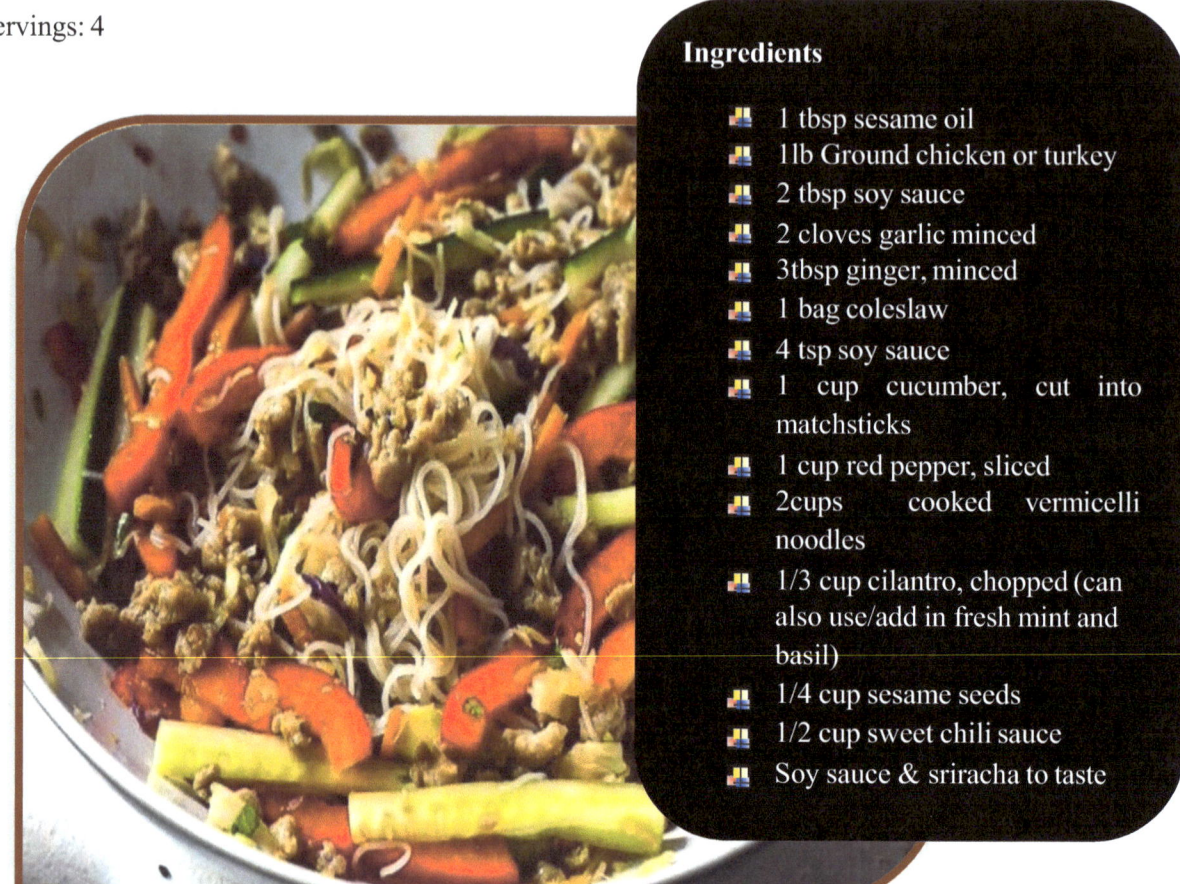

Ingredients

- 1 tbsp sesame oil
- 1lb Ground chicken or turkey
- 2 tbsp soy sauce
- 2 cloves garlic minced
- 3 tbsp ginger, minced
- 1 bag coleslaw
- 4 tsp soy sauce
- 1 cup cucumber, cut into matchsticks
- 1 cup red pepper, sliced
- 2 cups cooked vermicelli noodles
- 1/3 cup cilantro, chopped (can also use/add in fresh mint and basil)
- 1/4 cup sesame seeds
- 1/2 cup sweet chili sauce
- Soy sauce & sriracha to taste

Directions:

1. Heat sesame oil over med-high heat in a large skillet. Add ground chicken and 2 tbsp soy sauce, cooking for 2-3 min. Add garlic and ginger, then saute for 7-8 min until chicken is fully cooked.
2. Remove chicken from pan and add coleslaw and 2 tsp soy sauce, sauteeing for 2-3 min until slaw is slightly wilted. Meanwhile, cook vermicelli noodles according to package directions (usually takes 2-3 min in boiling water).
3. Add sweet chili sauce to 4 medium-sized mason jars. Divide chicken among jars, then coleslaw, cucumber, and red pepper. Top with vermicelli noodles, fresh herbs, and sesame seeds. Add soy sauce and sriracha if desired.
4. Jars keep in fridge up to 5 days.

Items You Always Want to Have in Your Pantry

When it comes to cooking quickly, stocking up your pantry with the right staples and equipment can go a long way towards helping you feed your family without having to slave over a hot stove for hours or spend a fortune. Here are some of the items you should always have on hand for quick, easy and cheap meals.

Pasta

This is a versatile food that can be used on its own or in other recipes. Italians have hundreds of sauces to add flavor to these humble little items made out of flour, eggs and oil. Use in soups, stews, salads, and on its own. Use spaghetti or one of the wonderful shapes the kids will love, like butterflies or twists. And of course, elbow macaroni is perfect for homemade mac and cheese, or macaroni salad.

Noodles

Closely related to pasta are egg noodles, which are great with dishes like stroganoff and chili if you don't want to serve it with rice. There are all kinds of Asian-style noodles as well, such as soba, udon and buckwheat. Even ramen have their place in a busy kitchen, as long as you don't use too much of the ultra-salty seasoning packets.

Rice

Rice offers an amazing array of tastes. White and brown rice are musts for the house. Parboiled is perfect for Mexican food. Jasmine rice is great with Asian food. Arborio and short-grain rice are perfect for risottos.

Tuna Packed in Water

Tuna packed in water can be eaten hot or cold. Go for the solid white albacore versus the chunk light, which can be very watery. You can buy eight cans of solid white cheaply at your local warehouse store for a fraction of what you would pay per can in the supermarket.

Want a real taste treat? Look for the gold cans of Bumble Bee Prime Fillet solid white. You can usually get six cans at the warehouse club for a reasonable price if you want to use the tuna as a featured entrée in an impressive dish such as tuna cakes or tuna Caesar salad.

Canned tuna is perfect for sandwiches, salad, tuna casserole, stuffed peppers, stuffed mushrooms, and more. Tuna is high in protein and low in calories and is a filling way to feed your family.

Eggs

Eggs are extremely versatile. As long as no one in your house is allergic, you can whip up dozens of meals in a matter of minutes. Try scrambled, poached, fried, over easy and soft or hard boiled. Make omelets, frittatas, quiches, French toast, pancakes, crepes and more.

Beans

Canned beans and legumes that have already been cooked are ideal for quick and easy recipes. Look for low sodium varieties of red and white kidney beans, pink, black and pinto beans, and chick peas.

Canned Vegetables

Not all canned veggies hold up well in salted water, but two that you should always have on hand for salad are beets and corn. Rinse well before serving and toss in your salad. Or, pickle the beets slightly with some white vinegar before serving as a side dish.

Frozen Vegetables

These are frozen at the peak of freshness on the farms and can be added to stretch any meal. Some frozen vegetables, such as cauliflower and broccoli, can be a real time and energy saver with a minimum amount of waste.

Fresh Fruits and Vegetables

Buy from your local farmer's market in small amounts you know you are going to use. They will have fewer pesticides on them and be riper and tastier than what you find in the supermarket.

Potatoes

White and sweet potatoes make an excellent accompaniment to a range of meals. You can keep it simple and cook them whole in the microwave, or make boiled, mashed, fries, hash browns and more.

With these staples in your pantry, there will always be something quick and easy to cook for dinner.

Kitchen Gadgets to Speed Up Your Cooking

There are literally thousands of kitchen gadgets available, from the humble to the gourmet. The right tools in the kitchen can really save you time and money. Here are some must-haves.

* A Good Set of Measuring Cups

These are essential if you want your recipes to turn out right, especially when baking.

* A Set of Measuring Spoons

These are also essential, for the same reason.

* A Kitchen Scale

This is ideal for measuring ingredients by weight. It can also help with portion control if you are on a diet. Don't guess at how much three ounces of meat is — measure it accurately.

* A Good Set of Mixing Bowls

Buy them in various sizes from small to large.

* Hand Mixer

This makes mixing everything from eggs to muffins a breeze.

* Salad Spinner

Wash your lettuce, give it a spin, and the centrifugal force will remove the water so the salad will be ready to put in a bowl. Tip out, add dressing, and toss to serve. You can also use it to drain pasta.

* Hand Chopper with a Plunger

This is perfect for you and your children to dice fruits, vegetables, cheese and so on without having to worry about cutting your fingers. Just push down on the plunger several times until you have the right-sized pieces for your recipe.

* A Mandoline Slicer

This will allow you to slice vegetables quickly according to your desired thickness. Put the handle on the thing you wish to slice so there is no risk of harming your fingers. Set the thickness and start to slice. It's ideal for making sliced potato dishes, apple pie and more.

* A Food Processor

A food processor will slice, dice, chop, grate, pulverize, and more, depending on what blades you have as attachments. The blender attachment can also help make smoothies, meringues and more.

* An Immersion Blender

An immersion blender is perfect for soups, stews and sauces. Instead of running the risk of burning yourself and splattering food everywhere in order to make your soup smooth (such as cream of mushroom soup), you just place the blender in the pot and start to liquidize all of the ingredients. Many of them have a measuring cup as part of the set. You can use it to whip up a smoothie in the morning, make scrambled eggs, and more.

* A Crock Pot

A crock pot, or slow cooker, will take some practice to master, but it is a great way to have a hot meal waiting at home for you and the family every night. Just follow the recipe and set the timer. It is also a great option in the summer .

. You won't want to turn on the oven or cook on the stove top when the temperatures soar. A slow cooker allows you to have a hot meal every night without heating up the kitchen and the whole house.

* A Foldable Colander

This sits flat in your cabinet so it does not take up a lot of space, and opens when you need to strain pasta, vegetables and so on.

* A 3-in-1 Cutting Board

Cut your items on the board and store them in the inserts until ready to use. One insert is a colander, the other a serving tray.

* An Egg Separator

This is ideal for all the times you need to separate your egg into yolks and white. Little chips of shell will be a thing of the past with the help of this useful gadget.

* A Cast Iron Frying Pan

It will take some time to break it in and learn how to cook with it, but it can last you years and never be thrown away because its non-stick surface is ruined, which is what happens all too often with modern frying pans. It goes from stove top to oven to grill and to table as well, making it very versatile.

Food Freezing Tips to Make Cooking Easier

Freezers are a modern marvel, a way of preserving many foods for several days to months so a busy household can have all the essentials on hand. Many foods you purchase from the freezer section of the store have been frozen right in the fields when the food is at the peak of freshness.

But let's start with foods you should NOT freeze.

* Raw eggs in the shells - they expand and crack.
* Hard-boiled eggs - they will get rubbery.
* Salad - lettuce and other foods with a lot of water in them are not meant to be frozen.

* Egg-based sauces, such as mayonnaise - they will separate and curdle.
* Dairy - milk, plain yogurt, low-fat cream cheese, cream and cottage cheese will all go watery and separate.
- Raw potato - it is also too watery to freeze. Cook it first, then freeze.

Getting the Most of Your Leftovers

- Now that you know what to avoid, let's look at what to do to get the best results from freezing your leftovers.

1. Always cool to room temperature

- Never put hot food in the freezer. It will raise the temperature and defrost foods around it. It will also get condensation on the inside of the container, which will make the food watery and unappetizing.

2. Freeze your food at the peak of freshness

- Don't freeze leftovers that are two or three days old just to try to salvage them. Freeze them on the same day you have cooked them so they are at their best. If you know you and your family really don't like to eat leftovers the next day, parcel them up into homemade TV dinners.

3. Use proper freezer containers

- Preserve your foods properly in freezer containers with a tight-fitting lid to retain freshness. Handle with care so nothing cracks when the containers are frozen.

4. Freeze into sensible portions

- Make single meals, or enough for a family of four, not twelve servings in one container.

5. Use freezer-friendly labels

- Use labels that will stick to your containers and hold up against the cold. Write clearly. Note the name of the recipe and the date it was frozen. Most frozen food should be eaten within three months, and not beyond six months.

6. Don't refreeze food

If you have bought a turkey, for example, keep it frozen until 24-36 hours before you are ready to cook it. Don't thaw and refreeze a raw bird. Thaw in the refrigerator to ensure even thawing and minimal bacterial growth. Once it is cooked, it is fine to freeze the meat.

7. Pack your freezer

A refrigerator runs most efficiently when there is space between the food to let the cold air circulate. A freezer works in the opposite way. A packed freezer is more efficient to run and more economical. Cook, make, and freeze recipes in batches, or fill your freezer with staples such as loaves of sliced bread and frozen vegetables.

8. Wrap or bag up your proteins when you get them home

If you are buying meat in advance, take it out of the store packaging and wrap it well. Or, place in a plastic bag you can seal tightly so you will avoid food being lost to the dreaded freezer burn.

9. If you live in a warm climate, bring a cooler and/or ice packs

This will help preserve the food and stop it from defrosting until you can get it home and into your freezer.

10. Purge your freezer every six months

Contrary to popular belief, freezing does not completely kill bacteria. Cooking at a high temperature will. Check your freezer contents and throw away anything older than six months, or anything which look suspicious.

Getting the Kids to Help with the Cooking

Home cooking when you are in a rush can be really stressful if you try to do it all yourself. But if your children are old enough to help, it's time to enlist them into the wonders of cooking and preparing food.

Safety First

The most obvious issue is safety in the kitchen. Children should not use sharp knives. They should always wash their hands well before engaging in any meal preparation. They should have an apron for their clothes and a work station away from any hot oven or stove with the burner on.

Invest in the Right Equipment

Be sure to have kid-safe mixing bowls and measuring cups. Also consider getting a chopper with a plunger. All they have to do is put the food under it and press down with both hands.

Make It Fun

Teach them fun and interesting things as you cook. Kids love to explore and learn.

Cook Their Favorites

Most children love pizza, pasta, burgers, meatloaf, and so on. They can help learn how to make all of these things. Have them help you roll out the pizza dough, or make English muffins or French bread pizza. Get them to help you toss the pasta with sauce, cheese and olive oil.

Let them roll up their sleeves to get messy with burgers and meatloaf. Use the plastic burger-forming shapes to get the children to make the burgers ahead of time, so all you have to do is defrost them.

For meatloaf, they will love to knead in the egg, spices, bread crumb, tomatoes and olives if you use them. At the end of the meal, have them help you make meatloaf sandwiches for the next day.

Create Stunning Salads

In addition to using their little chopper, the kids can tear lettuce into a salad spinner, wash the salad, and then spin to get all the water out.

. Create Delicious Desserts

Every child loves desserts. Keep control of what you eat by making them at home. You can cook quick microwave cakes, or bake a pie in the oven. Have the children roll out a pie crust — every child loves Play-Doh.

Bake cookies. Let them make mini fruit tarts with whipped cream. Try a bread pudding. Make muffins and cupcakes. Have them help cut up fruit for all kinds of desserts. Just remember to let fruit cool thoroughly if you cook it so it does not burn young mouths.

Create Healthy Breakfasts

While you are in the kitchen preparing dinner, or washing up afterwards, the children can help you get a head start on the next meals of the day. Scramble some eggs. Add cheese if you wish. Cook and crumble some sausage or bacon. Put it all together into a flour tortilla and wrap in waxed paper. You will have heat and eat breakfast burritos you can even take with you as you run out the door.

Try French toast you can heat and eat on the go, or French toast sandwiches with your favorite fillings, such as ham, cheese, Nutella, peanut butter, and so on.

Organize Brown Bag Lunches

If you and the family brown bag it every day, get a jump start by making them up the night before. The kids can lay out the bread, add mayo, mustard and so on, and layer the ingredients as needed. Make the sandwiches fun by letting the kids cut them with cute cookie cutters. You can eat the rest once the shapes are cut out.

There are lots of ways children can help in the kitchen. Start them off young and be patient and ready for messes. Over time, their skills will definitely improve, until they will be a real help in the kitchen and hopefully have developed a love of healthy food as well.

. You won't want to turn on the oven or cook on the stove top when the temperatures soar. A slow cooker allows you to have a hot meal every night without heating up the kitchen and the whole house.

* A Foldable Colander

This sits flat in your cabinet so it does not take up a lot of space, and opens when you need to strain pasta, vegetables and so on.

* A 3-in-1 Cutting Board

Cut your items on the board and store them in the inserts until ready to use. One insert is a colander, the other a serving tray.

* An Egg Separator

This is ideal for all the times you need to separate your egg into yolks and white. Little chips of shell will be a thing of the past with the help of this useful gadget.

* A Cast Iron Frying Pan

It will take some time to break it in and learn how to cook with it, but it can last you years and never be thrown away because its non-stick surface is ruined, which is what happens all too often with modern frying pans. It goes from stove top to oven to grill and to table as well, making it very versatile.

CONCLUSION

You can immediately start intermittent fasting for weight loss. You can follow either a weekly fasting interval or a shorter fasting duration. In the former, you abstain from eating your food for up to 24 hours one day a week. The second option allows you to fast for a lesser number of hours (say three to six hours) but more times weekly (two to three days in a week).

It is really up to you to find the intermittent fasting plan that will work best according to your needs. This is what sets it apart from the rest of the diet methods and plans. You can customize your fasting to fit your lifestyle. This is, also, what makes it more effective in burning your body fats to lose weight. The method does not tie you to any stringent protocol. It, therefore, increases your chances to succeed.

Intermittent fasting for weight loss is a simple method to burn body fats naturally. You work with your body by introducing healthy changes in your eating habits. As you retrain your appetite to distinguish what is real hunger from what you only feel like hunger, you lose your excess weight easily and quickly. Before you know it, fasting has already become part of your healthy routine.

Intermittent fasting isn't going to be for everyone but if you're serious about getting some real results then this will definitely boost them. Everyone should still learn the basics of a healthy diet and exercise program. You can definitely work out on your fasting days to enhance the fat loss but it will be extremely difficult for many to muster the energy to do so. Overall just make sure you plan ahead prior to your fasting day as it will be instrumental in your success with the program.

www.ingramcontent.com/pod-product-compliance
Lightning Source LLC
Chambersburg PA
CBHW041316180526
45172CB00004B/1115